MAGICAL
HERB
COMPENDIUM

About the Author

Aurora is an herbalist, aromatherapist, British Traditional Witchcraft high priestess, and registered nurse who has been using herbs and aromatherapy to heal people since 1990. Aurora studied with herbal teachers across the country, including two years with Matthew Wood and more than three years with Dottie Running Horse, a Dakota medicine woman. Visit her at Aurorasmagicalrealm.com.

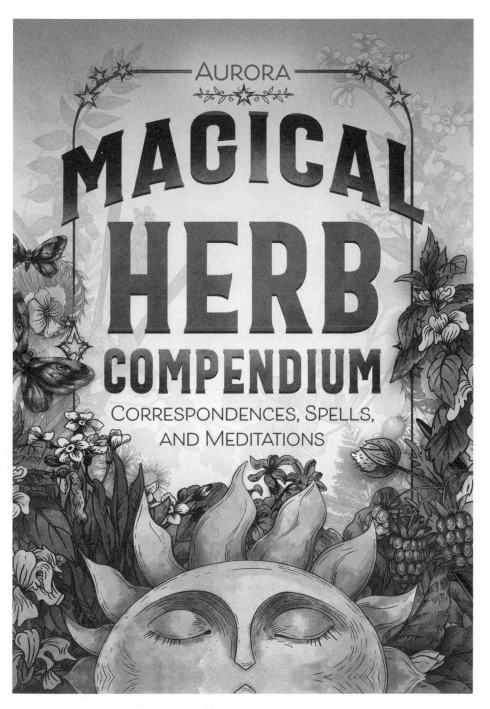

AURORA

MAGICAL HERB COMPENDIUM

CORRESPONDENCES, SPELLS, AND MEDITATIONS

LLEWELLYN PUBLICATIONS
Woodbury, Minnesota

First Edition
First Printing, 2023

Book design by Christine Ha
Cover design by Shannon McKuhen

Photography is used for illustrative purposes only. The persons depicted many not endorse or represent the book's subject.

Llewellyn Publications is a registered trademark of Llewellyn Worldwide Ltd.

Library of Congress Cataloging-in-Publication Data (Pending)
ISBN: 978-0-7387-7495-4

Llewellyn Worldwide Ltd. does not participate in, endorse, or have any authority or responsibility concerning private business transactions between our authors and the public.
  All mail addressed to the author is forwarded but the publisher cannot, unless specifically instructed by the author, give out an address or phone number.
  Any internet references contained in this work are current at publication time, but the publisher cannot guarantee that a specific location will continue to be maintained. Please refer to the publisher's website for links to authors' websites and other sources.

Llewellyn Publications
A Division of Llewellyn Worldwide Ltd.
2143 Wooddale Drive
Woodbury, MN 55125-2989
www.llewellyn.com

Printed in the United States of America

Disclaimer

Please note the information in this book is for the pursuit of maintaining the history of the plants' spiritual uses. There are toxic plants written about in this book that are for information only. Please do not use these plants unless you have a complex understanding of the toxicity and dangers associated with them. Please seek out the experience of a physician when taking herbs with other medications because there may be contraindications that are not understood at this time with the complexity of an individual's disease process. The advice in this book is not meant to replace the care of a certified professional, and readers should take utmost care when performing rituals, especially those that include bodily fluids.

CONTENTS

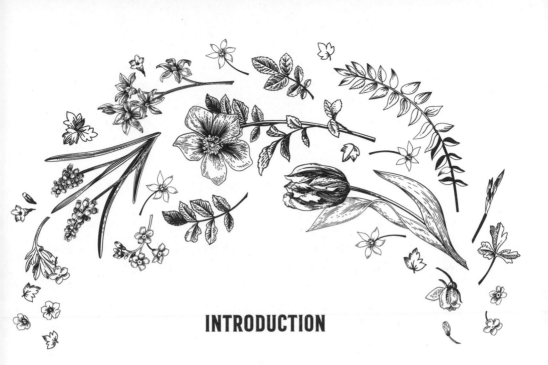

INTRODUCTION

This book is a lifetime in the making. It started when I began asking why the plants did what they did and when my grandmother told me the stories of her childhood with her Native American grandfather, who taught her about herbs, or her time in the Panama Canal. She often only knew the Native American or Spanish names of the plants, and she did not remember all of the information she learned.

In my journey, I have tried to recapture lost information from my Native American heritage, as well as gather information that is spread out in centuries-old books, which include not only herb books but folk histories, grimoires, and translations of hieroglyphs. One of my favorite plants, which I wrote about in this book, is the mandrake root (*Mandragora officinarum*). It is an herb that has been written about here and there, with a lot of good information already available on it, but I stumbled upon an obscure book on Romanian history that had a whole chapter on the mandrake root. It was information that I had not seen before, which gave a whole new depth to how this root is used. These kinds of finds are rare, and I have tried to add as much old and hard-to-find lore as I could so that it was not lost.

While capturing the old information, I also realized that I needed to add my own experiences to this book so that people can see different ways to use the herbs. Some of the herbs I have in this book have little written lore about them. Another one of my favorite herbs is wild bergamot (*Monarda fistulosa*), or sweet leaf. I learned about this plant first from my herbal teacher Matthew Wood and then learned more about its spiritual properties from Dottie Running Horse, a Dakota shaman and medicine woman I became friends and studied with. Most of the lore on sweet leaf is oral and, except for Matthew Wood's books, has never been seen before in print. As I studied this plant, I also realized that it was the plant that my great-great-grandfather used to cure my grandmother's migraines, which she only knew the Indigenous name for. My grandmother told me that her grandfather used to warm the fresh plant in water, place it on her forehead, then cover her forehead with a washcloth to relieve her headaches. So, life and its magic came full circle as I rediscovered my family's heritage with the plant people. Because of all the oral lore that I learned about plant magic, I decided to share it here so that the information is not lost in the sands of time. To me, passing on this information is one way to honor our ancestors. Because of this, I added the stories from Dottie Running Horse, as well as my own experiences with it and my research of the plant. I am honored to be writing the stories of my elders here and the stories of the plants that have taught me through the years. Enjoy their lore and their magic because, as they become a part of you, their wisdom will continue to live on and teach the next generation of medicinal and spiritual healers.

About Me

I started my herbal and spiritual path when I was quite young. I was one of those witches who learned how to use herbs to heal people as a child from my grandmother; she also taught me how to dye rocks and cloth using berries or leaves. She knew about many plants but did not know their Latin names and only had stories of how a plant could cure headaches or deep wounds.

I began using plants for magical purposes in the 1980s. At that time, there was not any information published that could be accessed online or that I could find in my local bookstore, so I spent hours at the public library; I ordered archived texts to read, and I spent many hours hand-copying the herbs and what they were used for. I also started collecting what I could from the only New Age shop within fifty miles. In the nineties I joined a magical group in upstate New York, and I started making some of the arcane recipes I had read about, including incense and tea, to sell at the local Pagan store.

When I moved to Minnesota, I went to nursing school and became a registered nurse. I started learning more about the magical use of herbs, and my thirst for knowledge drew me to learn not just the magical side but the medicinal side as well. I started training with local herbalists, such as Matthew Wood, and then I joined the Minnesota Herbalist Guild, where I was exposed to many amazing teachers who taught me even more about the medicinal side of herbs. I continued my studies and joined the American Herbalist Guild, a national herbal organization, and traveled across the country to national conferences to learn from more teachers about the magical and medicinal properties of herbs and resins. At some point in this journey, I started teaching classes on the magical and medicinal properties of plants, began writing about herbs in a publication called the Minnesota Pagan Press, worked part-time in a local herb/bookstore called Present Moment, and started a private herbal practice. A few years later, I became a professional herbalist in the American Herbalist Guild and eventually taught at several conferences on the medicinal properties of herbs. I have also trained to become an aromatherapist and flower essence practitioner, even traveling to Europe to take advanced classes.

I have trained with some of the greatest herbalists and natural healers in the world. Most of my training took place in the United States, but I have trained in South Korea, England, and France for my craft. I have had a natural healing practice for over twenty-five years where I have used plants to treat people for both physical and spiritual ailments. My magical credentials include being a Wiccan high priestess in a British traditional path for over twenty-five years, and I often speak at national or international conferences and festivals on how to use herbs to heal the mind, body, and spirit, as well as how to use them for magic.

How This Book Is Organized

This book is set up to give you the ability to instantly dive into the herbs and learn about how to use them in your magical practice, as well as provide you with more detailed information as you need it.

Chapter 1 briefly discusses the history of magical herbalism as we know it from ancient manuscripts, hieroglyphics, and cuneiform tablets. This chapter also introduces the doctrine of signatures, which is how we can observe plants in nature to determine what they can be used for in magic.

Chapter 2 teaches about wildcrafting and tells you how to harvest plants from the wild, including the tools that you will need to collect them, how to process the plants, and how to store them.

Chapter 3 details different ways to use herbs to make magical formulas and gives you some basic ways to make magical preparations. It also explores the items you will need to create an herbal apothecary.

Chapter 4 is the compendium of herbs, and each herbal monograph will show you how to use the herb, detail the deities and planet associated with it, and share a story of how I have used the plant in the past.

In chapter 5 there are incense, infused oil, tisane, and salve recipes. Some are given as examples, and others are recipes that I have used with good outcomes.

The appendix is a quick reference guide for you to find the herbs you need in order to put together a magical spell for a certain cause.

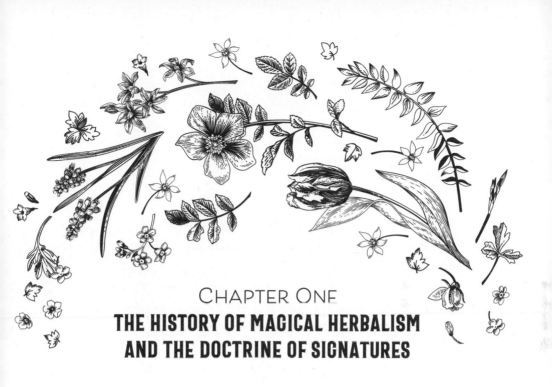

CHAPTER ONE

THE HISTORY OF MAGICAL HERBALISM AND THE DOCTRINE OF SIGNATURES

We don't really know when the first person put the first aromatic plants on the smoldering coals of a fire as an offering to their gods, but using herbs in spiritual practices was done long before it was written about. Many of the original rites and offering practices were passed down via oral tradition and were only written about years after they were in customary practice. We do not know how long these plants were used before books and other documentation were written, but what we do know comes from what was written on these tablets, on those scrolls, and in those books. In the following sections, I will attempt to create a timeline based on the information we can find from the periods and the people who wrote about the use of plants, even hundreds of years after the events first happened.

Sumerian

One of the things we do know about some of these ancient societies is that they traded herbs, spices, and resins between them, and these trades were documented. Sumerians are some of the first people to document the herbs and spices that they traded on cuneiform tablets. In addition to merchant records, there are a few recipes and details of medicinal preparations and resins used as offerings. Tablets from around 2963 to 2031 BC talk about offerings to Inanna, a Sumerian goddess of love, justice, and fertility, in heroic poetry; some of the herbs offered to her were frankincense and cedar.

Egyptian

The Egyptians documented evidence that they used resins and herbs as magical offerings, in spell work, and in the mummification process starting before 1473 BC. Many of the recipes were documented on papyri that were buried in tombs with mummies, often with the resins or offering blends in jars next to them to carry with them on their travels to the afterlife. Many of these recipes can be found in the works of Edward Budge, as well as other books that focus on Egyptian rites and rituals; many have modern substitutions for the hard-to-find items, such as asp tongue, in them. The Egyptians used mostly resins like frankincense and myrrh in their rituals and spiritual practices.

Indian

India has a rich history of using herbs, flowers, and resins in spell work aimed at healing and in love magic. Many formulas can be found in the Vedas, which are collections of hymns that were written starting between 1500 and 1200 BC; they provide guidance on various aspects of life, including worship of deities, healing, and attracting love. Many of the recipes are still in use today as ritual offerings and in long-standing traditions. Some of the herbs written about in the Vedas include resins such as gugal, sandalwood, and flower petals, which can be mixed with flour or common household items. What I love about the Vedas is that a lot of the traditions they detail are still being used to this day in sacred rituals.

Chinese

There is herbal information in Chinese texts dating back to the Han dynasty, which was between 202 BC and AD 220. Most of this information is more medicinal in nature, but it also has a lot of spiritual information, such as incense recipes for worship. Most of the herbal information in the Chinese texts is from China, but some of it is originally from Korea or Japan, as these countries are in close proximity and share Buddhism as one of their main religions. Herbs that were used for spiritual practices include sandalwood, resins such as frankincense, and aloeswood.

Greek

The Greeks developed their own system of medicinal philosophy to treat disease using a humor system. Many of their rituals, including the day-to-day worship of their deities, that were documented used herbs, oils, and resins. They burned large amounts of incense and gave many offerings, both to their private deities and to the deities of their leaders. The Greeks were heavily influenced by the Egyptians' use of herbs and resins in spiritual matters and often adapted early Egyptian recipes to fit the Greek deities. The Greeks used resins such as frankincense as well as cedar.

A Note about Resins

Most cultures used resins for incense and as offerings to the gods, all the way back to the Sumerians. Later cultures added woods and flowers that were growing around them to create more complex blends that they felt were appropriate to offer to their gods. We can take this historical information and let it inspire us to create an herbal magical practice that is local to where we live and that aligns with our chosen deities.

The Doctrine of Signatures

A long time ago, when I was just a girl, my grandmother taught me the importance of paying attention to the things around me. She taught me to watch the wind as it blows in the trees because it can foretell a change in the weather. She taught me to observe how the ocean swells at different times during the moon's cycle and how to decipher the stars in the night sky. She also taught me how to look at the plants around us and how to see the wisdom that Mother Nature gives us on a regular basis. This is something that we as a people have forgotten how to do. We can learn so much if we just look at the world around us and just listen to what the earth is trying to tell us.

Before the advent of modern medicine, ancient healers understood that how a plant looked gave them clues about how to use it for both healing and magic. This system of looking at plants and their visual patterns to get clues about what spiritual or medicinal attributes they may have is called the doctrine of signatures. This art of looking at colors, textures, stem shapes, and growing habits to determine what the plants can be used for shows us each plant's true virtue in a way that is easy to understand—without writings or the internet. It allows us to use the simple art of observation and communing with nature.

Several famous physicians, philosophers, and magically inclined people have used and written about how to use the doctrine of signatures. One of the first two people to write about this system was Roman scholar Pliny the Elder (AD 24–79). Pliny the Elder's *Natural History*, finished approximately AD 77, consists of thirty-seven books that contain information on astrology, mathematics, zoology, botany, agriculture, pharmacology, mineralogy, precious stones, and more. *Natural History* is one of the earliest references to the doctrine of signatures, but Pliny the Elder's recommendations on which plants to use for different diseases are limited because during this time the Romans did not allow physicians to cut open cadavers in order to deepen their knowledge of how the plants healed disease. Pedanius Dioscorides (AD 40–90), a Greek physician, wrote a highly respected book called *De materia medica* between AD 50 and 70. This work, which consists of five volumes, was used as a basis for all of the herbal pharmacies for more than 1,500 years; it gives some details on the doctrine of signatures but focuses more on diseases and how to treat them.

During the late Middle Ages, Paracelsus (1493–1541), Giambattista Della Porta (1535–1615), and Nicholas Culpeper (1616–1654) were among the strongest proponents of the doctrine of signatures, and they wrote several books that gave deeper explanations of how to use this system. They are the writers who are often quoted when it comes to the doctrine of signatures.

Paracelsus was a German-Swiss physician, alchemist, and philosopher of the German Renaissance period focused on the power of observation; he married this observational ability with his philosophical beliefs that were based in Hermeticism. Hermeticism is a philosophical and mystical system based off the writings of Hermes Trismegistus. These writings, which were created from about AD 100 to 300, are theorized to have actually came from a series of mystical and alchemical writers who all wrote under Trismegistus's name during that period.

Paracelsus was well known for his writings, including *The Hermetic and Alchemical Writings*, as well as his theory of *similia similibus curantur,* or "like cures like." His works and teachings promoted the use of the doctrine of signatures.

Giambattista Della Porta, who was a student of Paracelsus, was an Italian scholar, playwright, cryptography expert, and astrologer who had a fascination with the occult. He wrote *Magia naturalis* and *Phytognomonica*, both of which deepened the doctrine of signatures theory. These books are full of symbolism and alchemical references to how the plants will create the magical or medicinal desired change.

Another early proponent of the theory was Nicholas Culpeper, an English physician, herbalist, and astrologer, who published *The English Physician* in 1652. This work put the doctrine of signatures at the forefront in English herbalism.

Many more writers followed these leaders; the apex of the doctrine of signatures was during the Renaissance, but as science grew, the belief in the mystical attributes of plants decreased, with many physicians dismissing the doctrine of signatures as incorrect.

I would disagree with the dismissal of the signatures from nature because, as we have found using modern scientific tools, there are chemicals in plants that produce certain properties or signatures. For example, plants with deep yellow roots were historically thought to help the liver and gallbladder. Science has since shown that some of these plants contain a chemical called berberine. Berberine has been proven to help with liver, gallbladder, and endocrine disorders, which supports the historical doctrine of signatures theory; this is one example of how science supports the doctrine of signatures.

While the historical writers of natural medicine and magic may not have had the same level of scientific knowledge as we do now, the fact remains that many of the conclusions they made have been borne out by advanced testing and other validation. In magic we need not be hampered by the chemical's attributes or what someone says a plant can be used for. We can use our imaginations to connect the physical attributes of the plants to the magical acts that we need to perform. Colors and shapes are symbols that connect us to the universe, and I believe these plant signatures may be more real than the current scientific theory.

How to Use the Doctrine of Signatures

It is easy to use the doctrine of signatures when wildcrafting or growing a plant for magical use. To use this system, you just need to observe a plant's natural form and make comparisons. This can easily be done when looking at the color of a plant or its flowers. For example, yellow flowers might mean that the plant is good for the liver or attracting wealth and happiness. Red flowers can be used for love or passion magic, pink flowers can be used to attract true love or to help with painful emotions, and orange-colored flowers are attractants that can be used to strengthen spell work and bring new opportunity. Blue flowers can be used to attract peace, promote healing, and improve psychic abilities. White flowers can be used to help find the truth or connect to divinity, and purple flowers increase the power of spells and help connect to the gods. Any green plant can be used for healing or to attract money.

You can also observe the shape and growing habit of the plant to determine its magical uses; this is particularly helpful in healing magic, and there are many easy associations. A plant with a heart-shaped leaf may be used for healing the heart or for love magic. Ground ivy, also called creeping Charlie, has leaves that look like ears or kidneys. It grows close to the ground and has many ropelike stems that creep everywhere, including through cracks in the sidewalk. Magically, ground ivy can be used for healing the ears or kidneys, but it can also be used to hear things that are being said when you aren't there, or it can be used as protection.

In short, the doctrine of signatures is a system of looking at the natural world and applying the code that nature has provided for us. By observing nature, we can learn how the universe works and changes over time. Observing plants in nature is best, but you can always look at pictures taken of plants in the wild to observe the colors, shapes, and growing habits of the plants you want to use for spiritual purposes. Using the doctrine of signatures in picking plants for your magical, herbal journey will only strengthen your spell work and abilities.

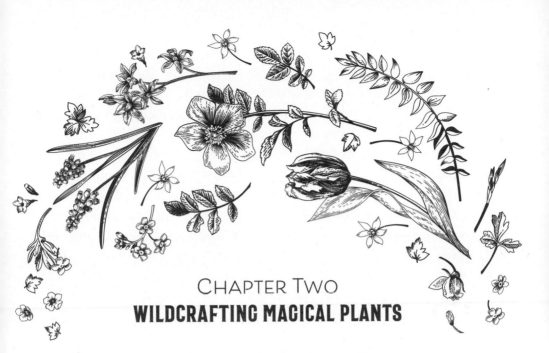

Chapter Two
WILDCRAFTING MAGICAL PLANTS

Wildcrafting is a common practice of going out into nature to collect plants, mushrooms, or resins or bark from trees. It is important when wildcrafting to make sure that you properly identify the item that you are collecting. There have been many cases of people misidentifying an herb or mushroom, eating it, and getting very ill. If you choose to collect plants in the wild, please go with someone who has experience identifying plants and wildcrafting; do not eat or use a plant you find in the wild before positively identifying it.

Basic Guidelines

There are some basic guidelines to follow when wildcrafting. The first and most important is to be careful where you harvest. You do not want to harvest plants from an area that was sprayed with poisons or gather them by a road where toxins and pollution might have contaminated them. It is also important that you do not harvest all the plants you encounter. A good general rule is to collect less than 10 percent of what you see; this will allow the plant to come back in the following years, meaning it should be there the next time you need to harvest it. If you are going to wildcraft plants, make sure you only take the part you need. For example, if you need leaves and flowers, just harvest those parts. Do not pull up the roots. Also know that it is traditional to leave a gift or offering for the plant spirit when wildcrafting. Common items to leave are coins, milk, bread, or honey. I like to leave jelly beans because the nature spirits seem to enjoy them and the sugar from the jelly beans will help nourish the plants as they dissolve. It is also traditional to ask permission of the plant before you harvest it. I can tell you from personal experience that the plants will answer you when you ask. I once went to harvest some red cedar for herb bundle wands, and the tree said no. I looked up, a bit confused, and then noticed tiny blue flowers in the branches. The tree was asking me not to harvest it so the flowers would get pollinated and produce cones and seeds, letting it reproduce. I also have been known to sing or play my flute to the plants as an offering before I harvest them. The most important offering is one that comes from the heart; it should also be something of value to the plant.

Tools for Wildcrafting Plants

There are several tools that you will want to have with you if you are going to wildcraft plants. One of these items is a trowel or shovel. This tool will be useful when you want to dig up roots or tubers, and it is easy to find short or camping shovels that easily fit in the trunk of a car. It is also helpful to carry a pair of hand pruners; this tool is helpful for separating branches from trees and cutting the branches into smaller pieces for transport. I always carry a small knife to cut nonwoody plants for harvest, remove resins from trees, or cut off seedpods.

It is also important to be prepared to transport your wildcrafted finds back to a processing area. For this, I bring plastic or canvas grocery bags. The plastic is perfect for carrying wet and dirty roots or juicy berries; the canvas is better for delicate leaves and flowers as it allows the plants to naturally dry as they are transported. I always have these items in the trunk of my car so I am prepared when I come upon an herb that I need to collect.

Preparing and Drying Your Harvest

Once you get your wildcrafted plants to where you will be processing them, you will want to clean them. To clean stems and flowers, you can simply rinse them off and hang them up to dry. When it comes to cleaning roots or rhizomes, you will need to wash the dirt off and make sure there are no rocks stuck in between the rootlets. Once the herbs or roots are clean, you can break them up by either chopping the roots or stripping leaves or flowers from the stems. If you plan to make a fresh-herb tea or tincture, use the plants immediately after cleaning them. If you are going to make an infused oil or salve, wilt the fresh herbs for a day to get the moisture out.

If you plan to store your harvest, you will want to dry the plants so the moisture is removed before you store them. The easiest way to dry herbs still on the stems is to hang them upside down in a cool, dry room. If dust, hair, or animal fur may be floating in the air, you will want to cover the plants with a large paper bag. Just put the plants in the bag, tie the top, and hang it to dry. You can also use an oven or dehydrator to dry your herbs. If you use an oven, make sure to set it on low (about 200 degrees Fahrenheit). Then spread the herbs out on a baking pan and place them inside the oven for a few hours until dry. Dehydrators can often be found at discount or thrift stores inexpensively and are wonderful to have on hand to dry harvested treasures. When using a dehydrator, dry the plants for two to three days until they are totally dry. Once the plants are dry, you will want to store them properly in glass jars.

Storing Wildcrafted Plants

It is important to store your magical preparations properly, keeping them dry and fresh so that you can use them when you need them. For medicinal purposes, herbs and roots can be stored for up to three years, but you can store herbs and roots to be used for magical purposes for up to six years. This is because with medicinal use, you are relying on chemicals in the plants; in magical workings, you are relying on the spirit of the plant. Resins last for years without losing much of their effectiveness and can be stored for as long as you need them.

The best way to keep your herbs, roots, and resins fresh is to store them in colored glass containers with lids in a cool, dry place. Using colored glass jars as storage is a cost-effective way to protect your precious herbs, resins, and roots. If you cannot get jars with colored glass, you can use clear jars, but make sure they stay in a cool, dark place, like a closet. If you do not have closet space available, you can put up a heavy-duty plastic rack and cover it with cloth to keep any light out.

It is especially important to label the jars that you store your magical plants in so that you can identify the plants later. You can use anything handy for a label. For years I used blue painter's tape because I had a lot of it left over after a painting project. You can also print some beautiful labels from your computer or a portable label printer. It is helpful to put the name of the plant on the label, as well as the day you bought or wildcrafted the herb and for what it is used. This way you can easily identify your herbs, roots, and resins as you learn to use them. Having a date on the label allows you to determine when you need to replace the plants. It is also helpful to organize them either alphabetically or by use. For example, if you wanted a section that had money-attracting herbs and another section for herbs to help attract love, it would make finding herbs for a formula easier.

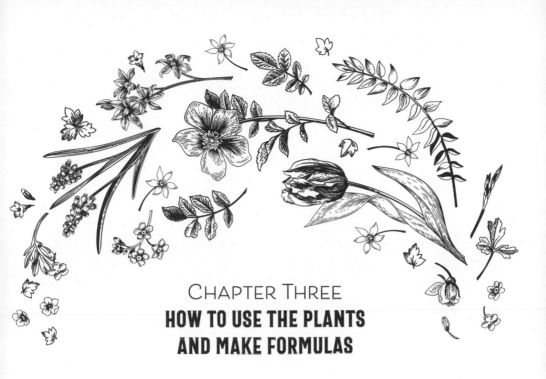

CHAPTER THREE

HOW TO USE THE PLANTS AND MAKE FORMULAS

This section has some vital information for the magical herbal practitioner, including different forms of the herbs and resins, how they can be used, and how to make different items with them. It also has a list of the tools you will need to make some of these formulas. This section will be very important as you grow your skills as a magical herbalist. I wrote this section to show you how easy it is to get started using plants and resins in your magical practice, and the list format will make it easy for you to get things as you need them. There are tips and tricks in each section, including how to get the highest quality herbs or resins and process them easily to add to a magical formula.

Herbs

Herbs as you buy them in the store are usually dried stems, leaves, and sometimes flowers. The consistency can vary, and they may be coarsely chopped or powdered. If possible, get your dried herbs chopped, which is often called cut, and sifted so that you can use them in several ways. If you buy your herbs powdered, it may be hard to identify them and use them for things other than incense. For example, powdered herbs do not make good teas as they tend to sink and do not integrate into the blend. It is also better to buy cut and sifted herbs, if possible, so that you will have the ability to grind them as needed. Grinding them as needed prolongs the life of the herbs; pre-ground herbs may be less potent than herbs ground yourself.

Herbs that are fresh should look close to their original color. If the plant is pale or does not smell as potent, it may not be as strong for your magical workings; you can sense the life force of the plant in its color and smell.

Flowers

I recommend trying to get fresh flowers, if possible, because dried flowers lose their potential quickly. This is because the volatile oils in them dry out rapidly on the petals. If you do buy dried flowers, buy whole flowers and make sure they have a scent to them. If they do not have a scent, they are probably not fresh. Do not buy flowers ground; they will have lower potency than whole ones.

Resin

Resins are gummy substances that are exuded from trees when they are injured. Frankincense and myrrh are probably the most well-known resins and have been used for thousands of years. They are becoming scarce in these times because of the overharvesting of the trees.

Different trees in the same family can have different grades, or qualities, of resin. For example, most of the frankincense we get in the United States is medium to low grade. The highest grade of frankincense is actually pale blue in color and mild in scent. It is expensive and hard to find unless you have a connection in the region where it is harvested.

Wood

Wood is the hard substance of a tree—the bark and inner wood. Wood has cellulose as the main skeletal structure, along with lignin and volatile oils, which protects the tree from insects. Many woods are not noticeably fragrant in nature, but when burned, they release a mild odor that supports a balanced magical blend. You can use the bark or twigs of trees to create incense, or you can use larger sticks to make magical tools such as wands. If you have woodworking abilities, you can make sacred bowls or statues from wood.

When using wood for incense, it should be ground right before it is used to get the most of its fragrance in the blend.

Essential Oils

An essential oil is the essence of a plant distilled down into a highly concentrated oil or waxy substance that contains all of the chemicals that create the scent of the plant. Thanks to this composition, they are a very powerful addition to your magical practice. Essential oils (except for lavender or tea tree oil) should always be blended with a carrier oil, such as almond or olive oil. Essential oils should not be used without diluting in a carrier oil because many of them can burn the skin when not diluted. When looking for an essential oil, make sure the bottle says "pure essential oil" or something similar. Perfume oils are made with natural oils mixed with synthetic chemicals that mimic a scent; they may say that they are an essential oil blend or contain essential oils, but they will not be pure. Perfume oils do not have the same spiritual abilities as pure essential oils. An example of a plant that comes in both an essential oil form and as a perfume is rose. Rose essential oil, or rose attar, is very expensive, hard to find, and can be several dollars per drop; a small dram bottle can easily cost more than one hundred dollars. In contrast rose perfume oil is very inexpensive (less than ten dollars per bottle at the time of this writing) and is easily found at any New Age store or holistic grocery store. Perfume oils can be used for magic, but be aware that since they contain unknown synthetic items, they may not work as well as a natural substance, or they may be toxic to burn in incense.

Teas and Tisanes

Teas are blends made with any tea (*Camellia sinensis*) plant; this includes black, green, and white teas. Tea can be added to any magical formula to strengthen it or ingested to help keep you awake. Tisanes are blends of herbs that are not from the tea plant. Teas and tisanes can be ingested, used as washes, put in spiritual baths, or used in cooking and can be used for medicinal or magical use. Drinking teas and tisanes is an excellent way to ingest magical formulas, especially for magical changes that you want to create inside yourself. For example, if you want to attract love, you may make a tisane with rose petals in it and drink it as part of your magical transformation. I have also made magical teas and added them to food so that the magic permeates the meal I am preparing. It is also easy to make a magically charged tisane and add it to your bath water, offer it to a deity, or use it to make soap or a magical lotion.

How to Make a Tisane or Herbal Tea

A tisane is actually an infusion of herbs in water, while a tea is an infusion specifically of tea (*Camellia sinensis*) leaves. In this book, we will talk mostly about making tisanes. To make a tisane, take equal parts of the herbs you want to use and blend them together. I usually recommend mixing a minimum of three different herbs together. To make a cup of tisane, take 1 teaspoon of the blend and put it in a muslin tea bag or a tea ball, then pour 1 cup of hot, but not boiling, water over the bag or ball, and let it steep for at least ten minutes.

Tinctures

Tinctures are liquids, usually alcohol, vinegar, or glycerin, that the vital components of herbs have been extracted into after sitting in them for a period of time. There are several ways to use tinctures to help with magical acts, and the liquids can be ingested or rubbed on the skin to create change. I have used tinctures for almost every piece of spell work. I have made tinctures that can help with divination, self-love, health, and money.

How to Make a Simple Magical Tincture

To make a tincture, take 1 cup of fresh herbs or ½ cup of dried herbs and put it in a quart Mason jar. Pour 80 proof vodka or apple cider vinegar over the herbs, making sure that it covers them. Cover the jar, put it in a sunny window for thirty days, and shake it daily. I like to start tinctures on the full moon. Once the herbs have infused their energies into the liquid, strain the herbs from the liquid. Compost the herbs or offer them to the earth, and then you will have a tincture of herbs to use in your magical practice. Take a few drops under the tongue to ingest the power of the herb, or rub it on your skin, poppets, crystal balls, or other items to make their magic stronger.

Incense

Incense can be a blend of herbs, flowers, woods, resins, and oils, or it can be a singular herb or resin. There are two main types of incense: one that you put on charcoal and one that has saltpeter or a combustible already in it.

It is better to make your own incense because you can control for purity, but also because you then have the ability to put energy into it as you make it. It is easy to add a few herbs and resins together with the proper intentions and then burn them on charcoal during magical acts. Making homemade incense sticks can be a bit harder, but there are shortcuts, such as buying blank incense sticks and adding oils and resins to them. Store-bought blends can be easy to use, but unless the incense is from a respected source, you probably don't know what additives are in it. Most commercially produced incense sticks have a higher amount of perfume oils put on charcoal bases. This produces scent and smoke for a low cost, but the sticks aren't made for your individual needs. You can get natural incense sticks, or you can make your own herbal blends, combining them under a full moon with intent; these will have a lot more power in them than commercially bought blends. Again, I encourage you to make your own incense for your magical workings. By making the incense, you manifest energy to create change and that intensifies the magic.

How to Make an Incense Blend

For the best balance of incense, combine at least one part each of wood, herb, and flower into a blend and mix it well while focusing on your intention. If you want to add an essential oil to the blend, do it after you mix all of the dried ingredients together and only add two drops of essential oil per ½ cup of blend. You can then burn the blend on a lit charcoal that is in a bowl filled with sand.

Infused Oils

Infused oils are carrier oils that have the energies and properties of plants infused into them. Carrier oils include almond, apricot kernel, coconut, or olive oil. They are neutral in nature and allow the scents of the plant materials to come through. I usually start making my infused oils under a full moon, but depending on the work you are doing, you may want to start yours on a dark moon. Beginning creation during a full moon is useful when attracting something to you, such as love or money. Making an oil during the dark moon is beneficial when you want to get rid of something, such as an ex-lover or bad luck. Making your oil under the sun/moon creates a strong magical oil that has the power of both the sun and the moon in it. Infused oil can be used to anoint tools, money, or people depending on what you want the oil to do. If you add a vitamin E capsule or use antimicrobial herbs or resins, these oils can last for more than a year.

How to Make an Infused Oil

The easiest way to make an infused oil is to start with dried herbs that have been cut and sifted; do not use powdered herbs as they will not blend with the oil. Put one part herb to 1 cup carrier oil in a glass pot, then put this pot in another pot that has a few inches of water in it. This creates a double boiler. Heat the pot with water on a stove top, and simmer the herbs in the oil for one to two hours, watching the pan with the water in it to make sure it never goes dry. Stir the herb and oil mixture every five minutes so that the herbs and oil blend well and don't burn on the bottom of the pan. Do not leave this mixture unattended during this time, and as you stir the mixture, put your intention into the oil. Once you have done this for at least two hours, strain out the herbs and put the infused oil in a glass jar with a lid to store.

Unguents

Unguents are semiliquid or oily salves that have medicinal or magical properties. A simple unguent can be made by infusing herbs in coconut oil or adding essential oils to coconut oil. You can also make an unguent by infusing herbs in olive oil and adding beeswax or cocoa butter to thicken it. Unguents are helpful when making scented magical formulas where the lingering scent works its magic.

How to Make an Unguent

To make an unguent, follow the directions to make an infused oil, using coconut oil that is solid at room temperature instead of an almond or olive oil carrier oil. You can also follow the infused oil directions as written and add a little beeswax or cocoa butter to the mix until it is thick at room temperature.

Herbal Wands

An herbal wand is a bunch of herbs that are dried and wrapped with cotton thread to bind them together. When people think about smoke purification, they usually think about cleansing sticks made from white sage, which is being overharvested in its native range and should only be bought if it's been ethically sourced, but there are other kinds of herbal wands that you can make from plants and trees that grow around you. I make herbal wands with local red cedar and herbs from my garden to make personal and powerful medicine. I use my herbal wands mostly for purification, but they have plenty of other uses. My favorite was an herbal wand for a fairy-style wedding; it was allspice bush, roses, lemongrass, and sprigs of lavender wrapped with white and purple cotton ribbons.

How to Make an Herbal Wand

The best way to make an herbal wand is to first harvest the herbs and let them wilt for one day, which decreases the water content in them. Once the herbs have wilted, bind them tightly by holding them with one hand and wrapping them with cotton embroidery or crochet thread.

These wands need to be dried, and I have found that the best way to dry homemade herbal wands is on the dashboard of a car, which quickly dries them, helping to prevent them from molding. I try to harvest the herbs for my herbal wands on days that astrologically align with the work I want to do. I then craft the wands the following day after setting the intention in the herbs.

Herbal Baths

Herbal baths are a combination of several things, including herbs and essential oils. Some traditions mix the herbs and essential oils with milk, others mix them with salt, and some people use both. I have found that making a dry bath for people to take home and use is easier than using liquid ingredients, which need to be bottled unless you are mixing them to be used immediately. Herbal baths are excellent for purification and healing, and they can be very powerful tools to add to your magical portfolio.

How to Make an Herbal Bath

For a dry bath mix, gather equal parts of powdered milk; sea salt; ground herbs, like rose petals; and a few drops of essential oils. Mix all of the ingredients together while concentrating on your intention, and then add it to a warm bath or store it in a glass container; this can be stored for up to a year in a cool, dry place. For a wet bath mix, simply use fresh milk instead of powdered milk and mix the ingredients together. Add the mix to a warm bath, or store it in a glass container in a refrigerator and use within three days. I make these on the full moon or dark moon depending on what they are being used for. Taking a magical bath during the full moon is useful when attracting something to you, like love, while taking a bath during the dark moon is beneficial when you want to get rid of something, like negativity or an ex-lover.

Gris-Gris Bags

Gris-gris bags are cloth or leather bags filled with herbs, crystals, oils, bones, coins, and sometimes charms for people to carry or place somewhere for magical acts. Gris-gris bags can be easily made using pre-made bags that you can buy at arts and crafts or Pagan stores and are easily customizable to fit your magical needs. I make these bags when needed, meaning I do not wait for a specific moon phase, because the crystals, the colors of the bag, or the herbs I put in them have the magical properties needed.

Tools Used in Magical Herbalism

There are many tools that you can use in the art of magical herbalism. These items should be dedicated to making magical formulas and should not be used to make dinner. Many of these items can be found at thrift or discount stores; my favorite glass bowl for making incense blends came from a thrift store for one dollar. When looking for items to use, look for damages like chips or cracks in the glass or peeling paint as these can get worse quickly when working with the natural oils in plants and essential oils. Try to connect spiritually with the piece before you buy it. I often close my eyes in the middle of a busy store and see if the universe will tell me if I should buy something as a magical tool. If the tool doesn't speak to you or you get the message to look for something else, listen and move on; often there is something that is meant to be used for your magical workings right around the corner. It will find you when it is time.

Mortar and Pestle

A mortar and pestle are critical when grinding herbs or resins. Make sure the inside of the mortar is not smooth; you want a slight texture on the side to help with the grinding. You can buy a small mortar and pestle in most New Age shops, but you can also find large ones at Asian or Hispanic grocery stores for less money because they are sold for cooking. It is better to use a large mortar and pestle when grinding resins because the increased surface area will make it easier to grind. A larger surface area will also keep cool longer than a small one. Grinding resins is hard work. A hack that makes it easier is to freeze the resins before you plan to grind them. When grinding resins, do not use a coffee grinder. Using a coffee grinder will heat up your resins, making them sticky. They will be difficult to remove from the coffee grinder, and your grinder will have a shorter life span as the oils in the resins will clog it.

Bags

Muslin bags make great tea bags and can also be used to make magical gris-gris bags. If you want to get fancy for magical bags, you can order sheer organza or velvet bags online or find them at most arts and crafts stores. Do not use the velvet or sheer organza bags for tea as the coloring agents used to make them may be toxic to ingest. It is helpful to align the color of the bag with the magical act you are performing. For example, if you want to attract money use a green or orange bag.

Bowls

I recommend using steel or glass bowls when you mix herbs and oils for magical or medicinal blends. Some plastic or ceramic bowls may release toxins or absorb the resins and oils, making them hard to clean or use for another magical blend. The bowls you use do not need to be fancy, but they do need to be dedicated to magic because, let's face it, frankincense-laced cookies won't taste good.

Utensils

Use stainless steel spoons, knifes, and whisks. Plastic or silicone utensils are hard to clean essential oils or resins off of completely, and they may leach toxins into your magical formulas. I have a kit in my magical room with a large spoon, a tablespoon, a fork, sharp knives, a rolling pin, bowls, and funnels; I keep it all in a plastic tote, which makes it easy to find and store my nonfood utensils.

Funnels

I suggest that people invest in a few funnels to make transferring items and potions into jars and storage containers easier. I have a set of stainless steel funnels to easily transfer liquids into bottles but also have a dedicated large canning funnel that helps pack herbs into glass jars for storage.

Grinder

You can use a simple coffee grinder for most leaves, stems, and flowers. If you want to grind roots, a coffee grinder will also do, but if you need to grind large amounts of roots at a time, I recommend investing in a Vitamix or another high-energy, strong grinder. You can often find them used online. As mentioned in the section about mortars and pestles, do not grind resins in a coffee grinder because it will be hard to clean and will decrease the life of the coffee grinder. You can use resin in a Vitamix if you freeze the resin first and then chop in short bursts so that the motor does not get warm. Resins are best ground in the frozen state in a mortar and pestle.

Silicone Molds

Silicone molds are helpful when creating the shapes of magical items, such as incense cones or magical bath bombs. I do not heat items in these molds because even though current science says they are food safe, I do not want to find out thirty years later that I used something toxic. This is my own quirk; you may feel comfortable heating in silicone, and that is fine.

Scales

In order to reproduce your best formulas, it is very important to measure and document the amounts of each item that you put in your formula by weight.

I have been making blends of teas and incense for more than twenty-five years, and I learned early to measure everything I put in the formula, even as I tweak it.

Recipe Book

You will want to store your recipes in a book or on your computer, especially when you find a recipe or formula that you want to create again. When I started creating magical recipes, I put my formulas in a blank book, which now has more than three hundred recipes in it. I have converted these recipes into files on my computer, but I have also had my computers die, and if I didn't have this hard copy backup, I would have lost many of my favorite formulas. Whatever form you choose to put your recipes in, make sure you keep updating it, and write down everything you make as you create it so that you have a record of it.

Storage Containers

When it comes to storage, I prefer using glass Mason jars for teas and incense mostly because they are reusable and easily washable, but there is also something oddly satisfying of seeing rows of glass jars on a shelf, filled with herbal goodies. If you use clear glass jars, you will need to store your herbs and resins in a closet or dark room in order to preserve the quality of the plant materials. If you have blue or brown glass jars, they can be out in the open because the color can block the light to a certain degree. If you need to create an area where you can keep your herbs covered, you can put them on a heavy-duty plastic storage shelving unit and use adhesive Velcro to help create a cover. To make this work, stick one side of the Velcro on the plastic shelf and the other side of the Velcro on a dark-colored cloth or tapestry, then connect the two Velcro halves together. This will create a cover for your herbs/resins, protecting them from light and extending their shelf life.

Labels

As I mentioned in chapter 2, it is important to create a label to put on your final product so that you know what it is. A label can be as simple as a piece of masking tape with the information written on it with a marker, but there are many other options, especially if you want to give your handicrafts out to friends and family or even sell them. You can go to an office supply store and create custom labels or borders for your labels, or you can create and buy labels from an online printing company. When I started out, I used tape and a black marker but eventually graduated to printed labels. On my labels I put the name of the herb or herbal blend, the date I made it, the astrological association (if important), and a *W* if it was wildcrafted, *D* if the material was dried, and an *O* if it is organic. You can structure your label however you want, but it is very important to label everything because after a few years, many leaves look similar, especially if they are already pre-cut and sifted for you.

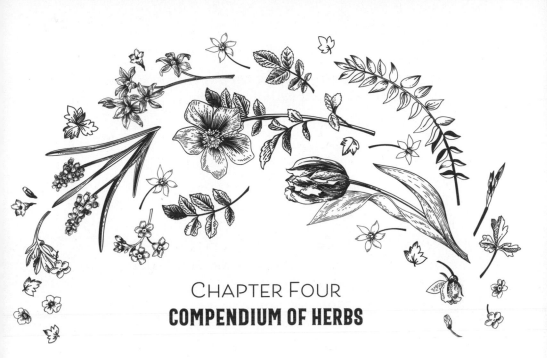

CHAPTER FOUR
COMPENDIUM OF HERBS

The herbs in this directory are herbs that I have used for both magical and medicinal purposes. I have spent decades learning how to use them, and my hope is that this directory, which includes stories of my personal experiences, will give both the beginner and the advanced herb user a good source to learn from. If you want to learn more about herbalism, I encourage you to study with your local herbalist so that you can discover how to identify the plants in the wild and learn more ways to use them.

It is always best to seek out organic herbs when you have to buy them. Do not wildcraft any herbs that have been sprayed with chemicals or poisons because they may cause health issues; plants found along roads have often experienced such contamination and pollution. If you plan to ingest any of these herbs, please ask your physician if they are contraindicated with any medicines or health conditions you have. Do not ingest any of the herbs that are listed as being poisonous. As mentioned, using herbs in your magical practice will not only increase the strength of your spells, but it will allow you to bring the power of nature into your life.

Aconite (*Aconitum napellus*)

Common names: Blue rocket, monkshood, wolfsbane, leopard's bane, woman's bane, mousebane, and Devil's helmet

Description: Aconite is a perennial that grows up to 3 feet tall. The root and stem are light green when young but get darker brown with age. The stem grows straight up, and the leaves grow around the stem opposite of each other. The leaves are dark green, glossy, and palmate in nature with at least three deeply toothed lobes. The flowers grow off the top of the stem and are medium to dark purple in color. The flowers look like hoods, which is how it got one of its common names. The flowers have an interesting inner structure that allows bees to crawl in, and as they do, the stamen, which is hammer shaped, rubs up against the bees' legs and pollinates the multiple stamens below. The seedpod is at the center of the flower, once the petals fall off, and there is a single small-sized seed inside of it.

Parts used: Roots

Cautions: This is a toxic plant; do not eat it, and do not burn it in incense. If you pick it fresh, wear gloves or wash your hands afterward. This is a strong herb that should only be used with the greatest of cautions.

Folklore and history: There is a lot of folklore about this plant. According to Maude Grieve in *A Modern Herbal*, aconite was created by Hecate from Cerberus's drool as he protected the gates of the underworld from Hercules. There is also lore about aconite being the poison that Medea tried to give to Theseus, who was her husband's long-lost son, when he came back to claim the throne. She was unsuccessful, and her husband, Aegeus, ended up dying instead, leaving Theseus the rightful heir. According to Greek myth, Medea learned her skills regarding herbs and poisons from Hecate.

One of aconite's common names is wolfsbane, and it is thought that this name was given to the plant because it poisoned the arrows used to kill werewolves. *Metamorphoses*, the epic poem written by Ovid in the eighth century, also talks of its poisonous abilities in one of its stanzas, and its ability to poison both human and beast has been well documented through the ages. In fact, there are many traditions around the world that speak of werewolves, the harm they cause, and how having monkshood for protection is helpful.

Spiritual uses: Protection, invisibility, protection against werewolves, worship of Hecate

Spiritual anecdote: This is a powerful herb that can be used for protection against werewolves, and if you don't believe in them, let me tell you a story I heard from my teacher Dottie Running Horse. She told me a story of a young man who boasted that he had killed a large buffalo when, in fact, it had died of illness and wolves had already started eating it. He took out his bow, shot an arrow, and nicked one of the wolves in the ear, so it came after him and bit him. The young man only had a small bite from the wolf because he continued shooting arrows, scaring the pack away. After this incident, the young man became agitated and scratching his head and back with whatever he could. One day he went to rub against a pine tree and got sap on his back. When he pulled away, several long hairs came out of his back. He continued to get hairy and agitated, and even started foaming at the mouth; he was sent to live on his own. Several warriors saw him in his traditional clothes, but he was covered with hair and ate carrion the same way scavenging animals did. The warriors went to kill him to put him out of his misery, but he could not be killed with normal arrows. To kill him, the warriors had to tip their arrows with aconite root poison. As with many of Dottie's stories about people who transformed into animals, it was really more of a spiritual transformation than a physical one.

Astrological association: Saturn

Deities, angels, or spirit associations: Hecate and Medea

Meditation: Sacred herb, protect me in my hour of need by keeping my enemies away from me.

Magical spell: Mix ¼ cup of ground dried aconite root in 4 cups of salt, then use this salt to put a protective circle around your home or work. This will also keep away werewolves in all forms. The salt blend can also be sprinkled on tools and crystals for protection as well.

Agrimony (*Agrimonia eupatoria*)

Common names: Common agrimony, church steeples, cockeburr, cocklebur, stickwort, and sticklewort

Description: This perennial grows up to 1 to 2 feet tall. Its reddish-black, creeping rootstock produces a hairy, erect stem that bears leaves that can be 8 inches long at the bottom of the stalk and up to 3 inches long near the top. The leaves are oblong-oval in shape, pinnate, and alternate along the stalk; they are toothed along the margins. The leaves and stems are deep green and have an odor similar to the scent of apricots. The bright yellow flowers grow on terminal spikes and are ⅜ of an inch long with five petals. The seeds are enclosed within a circular capsule of hooked spines.

Parts used: Dried aerial parts

Cautions: Should not be taken internally if constipated or if pregnant. Agrimony can affect prescription antidepressants, including selective serotonin reuptake inhibitors (SSRIs) and monoamine oxidase inhibitors (MAOIs), as well as anticoagulants, such as warfarin.

Folklore and history: This herb is named after Mithridates VI Eupator, king of Pontus, who was a famous herbalist. *Agremone* is a Greek word given to plants that were used to treat ailments affecting the eyes. Pliny referred to it as an "herb of princely authorities." The Anglo-Saxons, who called it *garclive*, applied it to wounds and believed it could cure warts and snakebites. Chaucer recommended *egrimoyne*, mugwort, and vinegar for "a bad back" and "alle woundes." During the fifteenth century, it was the prime ingredient of arquebusade water, a battlefield remedy for gunshot wounds, and it is still used today for sprains and bruises. It is an ingredient of spring tonics in many parts of Europe and a popular tisane in France. The whole plant yields a yellow dye. This attribute indicates that agrimony can be used for tension, inner torment, and hair problems, such as alopecia.

Spiritual uses: Magically, agrimony is an herb that can be used for protection, soothing tense situations, and liberation from negative relationships. Agrimony can be carried to ease or erase tension or obstacles when dealing with work or people.

Spiritual anecdote: A friend of mine had a run-in with her boss at work. She loved her job, but the problem caused her boss to increase her workload, as well as to talk badly about her behind her back. I had her carry a sprig of agrimony at work and put another under her computer. As of our last conversation, her boss had gotten a transfer to another department, her extra work started getting noticed, and she received a promotion.

Astrological association: Jupiter

Deities, angels, or spirit associations: Apollo and Hera

Meditation: Imagine a staff or large wand with the tip covered in bright yellow flowers, each flower having five petals. Each of these flowers is rotating clockwise like a fan. As you hold this vision in your mind, say: *Agrimony, stand firm with me and help me clear a safe path, free of obstacles and negativity. Help me get through these hard times and place me in the best situation possible.*

Magical spell: This herb is best used either dried or infused in oil. It is easily used by carrying it in a bag for protection against obstacles and negativity or by placing a few leaves where you want obstacles to be minimized, like under the computer at work. It can also be added to food, and the infused oil can be worn.

Angelica (*Angelica archangelica*)

Common names: Angelica root, root of the Holy Ghost, angelique, wild angelica, and dong quai

Description: Angelica grows 5 to 6 feet tall. Its biennial root is fleshy, spindle shaped, thick, and long. The color externally is gray brown, and it is whitish or yellowish white within and has a pungent smell, as does the entire plant. From the top of the root, a stem grows, which is purple, hollow, and fluted on the external surface. The leaves are bright green, large, borne on hollow stalks, and can grow up to 3 feet in length. They are bipinnate with lance-ovate, serrated leaflets with finely toothed margins. The flowers are greenish yellow, small, and numerous. They form umbels, which are grouped into a larger semiglobular grouping. These flower groupings grow on top of a hollow stem that shoots off the main stem. The flowers bloom in June or July and produce pale yellow oblong seeds, ⅙ to ¼ inch long, that have three ribs on the convex surface.

Parts used: Roots and stems

Cautions: None known

Folklore and history: According to M. Grieve in *A Modern Herbal*, in Pomerania and East Prussia, it was the custom until 1945 among the peasants to march into towns carrying angelica flower stems. They would sell them while chanting a song learned in childhood. The plant became linked with archangelic patronage of Saint Michael because it bloomed on his day, which is May 8. This flower is also associated with the Christian festival of the Annunciation, and because of this, it became connected with the ability to protect the holder against Witchcraft, enchantment, evil spells, and spirits that would do them harm. The root of the angelica plant was very protective—so much so that it was called "The Root of the Holy Ghost."

Spiritual uses: Communicating with spirits or the gods, repelling of Witchcraft and enchantments, protection, helping to create purity or restore innocence.

Spiritual anecdote: One of my herbal clients was having problems with a member of the spiritual community attacking him magically for committing a wrongdoing and lying about it. After I counseled my client on the importance of being honest, I performed a ritual, and one of the herbs I put in my client's bag was angelica root. It worked to ward off the negative magic. My client was then instructed to make amends with the person he wronged before the next sabbat, which he did. The curse/negative magic then dissipated over a short period of time.

Astrological association: Venus

Deities, angels, or spirit associations: Michael the Archangel and Aphrodite

Meditation: Imagine the large white flowers and say: *O plant of the angels, keep me safe as I walk in the darkness and light my way toward renewal.*

Magical spells: For protection, take a piece of this root, wrap it with red thread, and place in a bag to wear around your neck while chanting the plant's meditation three times. The whole root can be hung in a window for protection against negativity or Witchcraft, and the essential oil of angelica can be added to candles or made into a protective perfume.

Apple (*Pyrus malus*)

Common names: Crab apple and wild apple

Description: The crab apple tree can grow up to 30 feet tall, but it is usually found to be the size of a large bush or small tree (4 to 5 feet tall). The wood is gray and deeply furrowed or scaly; some mature trees have thorns on the branches. The leaves alternating up the stem can be up to 4 inches long. They are medium green and lance shaped with a finely serrated edge. One of the most beautiful parts of this tree are the flowers; they come in several pastel colors, including white, pink, and red. Each flower has five rounded petals with multiple yellow stamens. The fruit is round with a flat bottom that grows up to 2 inches wide. It can also be a variety of colors, including shades of red, pink, and yellow.

Parts used: Fruit and wood

Cautions: None known

Folklore and history: Our modern apples come from carefully cultivated crab apple varieties and can be used interchangeably for magical acts. There is mythology related to the wild apple, or crab apple, that goes as far back as the Sumerians. In the Sumerian story of Enki and Ninhursag, Uttu, who is Enki's descendant, was the last goddess to be seduced by him, and he did so by bringing her an apple and some vegetables. Luckily, Ninhursag intervened and the cycle of incestuous relationships ended. In *The White Goddess*, Robert Graves calls apples one of the "seven sacred Trees in the grove." When you cut an apple in half horizontally, you will see five seeds in a pentacle pattern. It has been a sacred fruit to use as an offering to many deities and is a sacred fruit that can be used in rituals and in beverage.

Spiritual uses: Fertility, healing, promoting love, and increasing psychic abilities

Spiritual anecdote: I had a friend who helped women who thought that they were infertile, and oftentimes we would team up. I would use herbs to help with any medical issues, and she would make them charms to help them conceive. One of the items she made for women who had a really hard time conceiving was a garland of dried apples slices, cinnamon sticks, and dried oranges on orange embroidery thread, which the women would then hang above their beds. The scent of these garlands was wonderful, and the magic of the fruits and cinnamon often helped these women conceive.

Astrological association: Jupiter

Deities, angels, or spirit associations: Aphrodite, Uttu, Gaea, Hera, Athena, and Abellio

Meditation: To help increase fertility, close your eyes, imagine a pink light surrounding your body, and say: *Apple, sacred fruit, help ensure fertility for me, and help me to conceive a child.*

Magical spell: The following is a spell to find true love; it is not meant to be used to attract a certain person, but a future love. Take a regular apple and cut it in half horizontally. Dig out a hole in the center of the apple large enough to put a tealight candle in it. Light the candle. As the candle burns, close your eyes and meditate on how you would like love to come into your life. First, envelop yourself with a pink light. This is self-love, and it must be accepted before you can move forward to true love. Concentrate on what you want true love to look like in your life. Imagine how it will be to feel love in your life and how it will make you a better person. Meditate on this for thirty minutes before extinguishing the candle. Perform this meditation daily, relighting the candle each time, until the candle burns out. When the candle is finished, bury the apple and candle in a protected location outside. Do this ritual once every full moon for thirteen months. At that point, true love should come to you.

Asafetida (*Narthex asafetida* or *Ferula foetida*)

Common names: Stinkweed, Devil's dung, and food of the gods

Description: This plant grows to be about 6 feet tall and has feathery, dark green leaves. The flowers are small and yellow and grow in a grouping that looks like an inside-out umbrella. Asafetida flowers in June, and after flowering, the seed capsule turns dark brown and contains small brown seeds. The part of the plant that is used is the gum, or resin, which is exuded from the roots of five-year-old plants. This gum has a most distinctive odor, smelling like slightly fishy, rotting onions. The entire plant has the resin's characteristic odor, but the root contains the strongest scent.

Parts used: Roots

Cautions: None known in therapeutic doses. If you do choose to use this herb, use it sparingly. I have known people with sensitive stomachs who are not even able to be in the room with an open jar of this herb. Not many stores carry this herb, but you can find it at most Indian grocery stores in the spice aisle.

Folklore and history: Asafetida is an interesting plant that is not often used due to its offensive smell and unusual taste, but it is an excellent medicinal and magical herb, and it has been used since the time of the Romans for medicinal, magical, and culinary purposes. The Romans used it medicinally to treat respiratory diseases and indigestion. They also used it for protection, to exorcise demons and spirits, for invisibility, and for purification. It was used in several pungent fish recipes, and it is still used today in some cooking to add a pungent onion flavor to lentils.

Spiritual uses: Exorcising demons and spirits, protection, and invisibility

Spiritual anecdotes: I only use this resin when banishing the most nasty and tenacious of spirits from people's houses. One such house was on a US Air Force base that had been built on a ley line; the spirits were so strong they had managed to physically push two people in the house (one almost down the stairs). A team of us managed to direct the spirits out of the house while burning some of this resin (of course the smell was so horrible; we all disliked it). I have a friend who puts some of this resin in salt and sprinkles it around her house whenever she feels she needs extra protection from harmful people or situations.

Astrological association: Mars

Deities, angels, or spirit associations: Kali, Shiva, and Lucifer

Meditation: All evil and negativity be banished from my presence, let it be known that this is a safe place, and no spirits or demons may return.

Magical spell: As mentioned, I use this herb to chase really nasty spirits or demons away. The best way to get the positive effects of this herb is to

mix it in salt and put it around your home as you say the plant's meditation. I rarely burn this herb in incense because it has a very strong odor
that is hard to clear. If you burn it, keep the windows open and make
sure you have good ventilation.

Ash, Prickly (*Zanthoxylum mericanum*)

Common names: Toothache bush, toothache tree, toothbrush bush, yellow
wood, suterberry, and northern prickly ash

Description: Prickly ash is a native North American shrub that grows up to
10 feet tall; it inhabits damp soils from Canada to Virginia and Nebraska.
The bark is smooth and gray with occasional lighter gray splotches; the
bark can be grooved in older trees. The branchlets grow up the stems
bearing two thorns up to ¼ inch long at each nodule. The leaves grow
alternately up the stem with five to eleven oval leaves that grow on each
end of the stem with a single leader leaf at the end. The leaves are 1 to 2
inches long and dark green on the top, but the bottoms are lighter green
due to the fine, white hairs covering the leaves. Small, yellowish-green
flowers grow in axillary clusters during April and May, before the leaves
appear; male and female flowers grow on different plants. The fruit is a
small, red berry-like capsule captaining one or more shiny, black seeds.

Parts used: Leaves

Cautions: None known

Folklore and history: According to some folk medicine texts and Indigenous healers, prickly ash was used to treat toothache pain because it has
a numbing action when chewed. The Native American spiritual lore that
I received from Dottie Running Horse was to put the bark shavings and
thorns along with tobacco in a red flannel bag to protect the wearer against
certain Great Plains spirits, who would cause travelers to get lost on long
journeys.

Spiritual uses: Protection (general), protection from getting lost, and removing spells and curses

Spiritual anecdote: I had a client who was a truck driver. He had some
medicinal issues, which I helped him with, but while driving he often
left the main road to go to some small diner to eat. He loved good food

and was willing to detour a short distance to get it. The only problem was that he tended to get lost on the way back to the highway. Now, this was before we had GPS mapping, so he relied on paper maps to get him to these places, and sometimes the maps were not updated to have all of the small roads on them. I gave him a prickly ash tincture to help with his medical issue but also gave him a small bag to carry in his truck with prickly ash shavings to keep him from getting lost, a piece of obsidian to help ground him, and a piece of rose quartz to bring him home safely to his wife and three children. During his next visit to me, he said that he thought his sense of direction was getting better because he was finding the diners and his way back to the highway easier.

Astrological association: Mars

Deities, angels, or spirit associations: Saint Christopher, Hermes, and Adiona

Meditation: For protection, say: *Prickly ash, use your powers of protection to keep me safe from harm and protect me from evil.*

Magical spell: For general protection, cut up a prickly ash branch into 1-inch pieces, including some thorns, or buy some dried prickly ash. Put the prickly ash, plus a piece of obsidian, in a red flannel or velvet bag and carry it with you.

Aspen, Quaking (*Populus tremuloides*)

Common names: American aspen, trembling aspen, and golden aspen

Description: Quaking aspen is a large tree that grows up to 80 feet tall. The tree's root system is an adventitious one, as new trees grow off new roots and are identical clones of the original tree. Each quaking aspen can live up to 150 years, but the network of trees in the connected root system can live much longer. According to the USDA Forest Service, the oldest known root system is in Utah in Fishlake National Forest. It is estimated to be 80,000 years old, weighs approximately 13 million pounds, and has more than 40,000 trees growing from it. The bark of the tree is pale gray with black, horizontal lines. The bark has the ability to produce food, even when there are no leaves on the tree, through photosynthesis. The leaves of the tree are oval and dark green with a light green vein through them. They turn golden yellow in the fall. The edges of the leaves are finely serrated, and the leaves are flat and hang on long stems, which is why they seem to tremble in the wind. The flowers are small, yellowish white, and grow on catkins at the edges of the branches. The seeds are very small and light brown in color.

Parts used: Leaves and bark

Cautions: None known

Folklore and history: The quaking aspen is a North American tree that was used by many Native Americans for food and medicine. There is some lore from the Dakota tribe I studied with about the leaves' ability to talk to the people to warn them of danger from evil wind spirits and to answer questions. It is said that the ancestors speak to the people through the leaves' trembling.

Spiritual uses: Immortality, knowledge, healing, and communication with the dead

Spiritual anecdote: I had a colony of quaking aspen trees in my yard in Robbinsdale, Minnesota, and when I had to make some major life choices, I would go and sit under the largest tree and talk to it. I would ask questions, and the trembling leaves would give me answers, but the tree did not only speak in yes or no answers. The leaves, as they fell in the fall, would sometimes create a picture, giving the tree the ability to send more detailed messages. Because the tree was connected to all other quaking aspen trees in the region, it was able to access a large spiritual bank of knowledge, and it helped me make some decisions that I may not have been able to make without it. It is a tree that can connect this world to other worlds and to our ancestors, and it is a powerful plant spirit.

Astrological associations: Pluto and Saturn

Deities, angels, or spirit associations: Michael the Archangel, Phaethon, Apollo, and Aura

Meditation: *Tree of the mother, tree of communication with my ancestors, help connect me with the truth; help me make the decision that will give me the best outcome.*

Magical spell: To promote a long life , plant a quaking aspen and place a gold coin and a letter with the name of the person who wants a lengthy life under the roots. Water the tree every day with blood meal mixed in the water for the first ten years of its life. Once the tree blooms for the first time, take the first catkin that falls and have the individual carry it. This catkin should give them a lengthy life as long as they carry it.

Basil (*Ocimum basilicum*)

Common names: American dittany, Saint Joseph's wort, witches' herb, and sweet basil

Description: Sweet basil is an annual that grows to be around 3 feet tall. The stems are square, and the leaves are medium green on top and grayish green on the undersides; they grow to be 1 to 1½ inches long. In late July or early August, the plant sends out a flower spike that produces flowers that grow in whorls around the stem; the flowers are small and white and have the same scent as the leaves. The seeds produced are small, dark brown, and easily collected to use the next year. The one thing that is most distinctive about basil is its scent. Basil has a distinctive camphor-clove smell that is hard to ignore. It is the defining characteristic in its identification.

Parts used: Leaves

Cautions: None known

Folklore and history: In John M. Riddle's *Dioscorides on Pharmacy and Medicine* and Galen's *On the Constitution of the Art of Medicine*, it was written that basil was believed to have a strong connection with invoking scorpions and that even smelling the herb could "bring scorpions to (into) the brain." According to E. A. Wallis Budge in *Egyptian Magic*, Egyptians and Persians revered this herb and used it as an offering to their gods and to their dead as they began their journey into the underworld. In some cultures, when a sprig of basil was accepted by a maiden, it was a sign that she accepted the love of the man handing it to her.

Spiritual uses: Basil has an association with passionate love, which means it can be used for lust magic. In fact, a passion-infused dinner using basil is one of the easiest ways to add magic to a relationship. Basil also has the association of luck and money; a sprig of basil is said to ensure good luck and fortune. In order to attract money, a sprig should be placed in your wallet or carried in your pocket after you have willed your intent into it. Make an infused oil with basil and pine needles to rub on candles and dollar bills prior to spending for money magic. Basil-infused oil can be rubbed on pulse points prior to job interviews. Basil also has a minor underworld association and could be used in rituals when invoking underworld deities or during Samhain. Basil incense burned at a Samhain ritual can encourage spirits of the dead to join the ritual.

Spiritual anecdote: I make an infused oil out of basil and pine needles with which I anoint candles, my wallet, and dollar bills. When making the oil, it is important to concentrate your intent of the magical working into the oil.

I once gave some of this oil to one of my friends whose car had broken down; he needed several thousand dollars for repairs. He put this oil on a twenty-dollar bill and spent it during the day. Two days later he got a credit card with a large enough limit to cover the amount due on his car, and three weeks later he got a promotion with a nice pay raise. I always keep a batch of this oil on hand for when money is needed for an emergency.

Astrological association: Mars

Deities, angels, or spirit associations: Zeus, Aphrodite, Anubis, Osiris, and Sekhmet

Meditations: For love, say: *Oh, basil, sweet basil, let your sweet scent attract my lover to me and make them desire me.*

For money, say: *Dear friend, green basil, let the money flow to me and be as plentiful as your seeds. Let the scent of money crossing my palm be as intense and as prolific as your sweet scent.*

Magical spell: To spice up your love life, you can use my simple method of making a tisane out of basil leaves. Just take 1 tablespoon of the dried herb and steep it for ten minutes in a cup of hot water. Once you've made and cooled the tisane, put it in a spray bottle and spray it wherever your love usually sits and on the bed. Your partner will be stimulated by the scent and attracted to the bedroom area.

Benzoin (*Styrax benzoin*)

Common names: Gum benjamin, Sumatra benzoin, and Palembang benzoin

Description: A tree native to Sumatra and Java, benzoin has leaves that are oval to lancelike in nature and grow in alternating pairs down the stem. The leaves are dark green on the top and silver gray on the bottom due to small silver hairs. The flowers, before opening, are oval in shape and, when opened, have four to five pink petals. The seed husk is green to light brown and globular in nature, while the inner part of the seed is white to light yellow in color.

Parts used: Resin and essential oil

Cautions: None known

Folklore and history: Benzoin has been used for thousands of years for both medicinal and spiritual healing. Benzoin gum is obtained by making triangular cuts in the tree from which the sap exudes and hardens on exposure to air. The first exudate forms almonds of benzoin followed by grayish-brown resinous lumps. These are compressed together into a solid mass. Benzoin is currently used in the perfumery industry as an antioxidant and fixative. Benzoin resin can be burned in open space in order to release its antiseptic properties, and it is one of the ingredients in church incense. Benzoin is the main ingredient of friar's balsam, a healing salve that was once widely used in Europe.

Spiritual uses: Purification, attraction, and prosperity; I use this scent primarily for purification, either as a blend with frankincense and myrrh or by itself. Its gentle vanilla-like scent is a nice addition to incense blends. Benzoin can also be made into an anointing oil to rub on the body or objects. I have also used this as an incense to help people who had a substance abuse disorder.

Spiritual anecdote: This is one of the resins in the three king's formula, which is a combination of frankincense, myrrh, and benzoin, and in several purification blends used by the Catholic church. One day, around Easter, I was working at Present Moment Herbs and Books, where I was an herbalist, and a Catholic priest came in wanting to buy pounds of benzoin resin. I gave our buyer the order and talked to the priest for a while. Even though he didn't go into exactly what he wanted the resin for, it seemed like, in addition to being used at Easter as a spring purification incense, it was to be used in some of their anointing oils. Of course, I made a note of this in my journal for the next time I needed to create a purification incense.

Astrological association: Sun

Deities, angels, or spirit associations: Inanna, Sekhmet, Anubis, and Ra

Meditation: Ancient resin, blood of life, purify me in my time of need so that I may be acceptable for (insert reason).

Magical spell: While burning incense of benzoin, imagine that the cloud of smoke embraces you and clears you of all negativities and everything you want to get rid of.

Betony, Wood (*Stachys officinalis*)

Common names: Bishop's wort, betony, and Betonica

Description: Wood betony has a deep, woody root from which square, green stalks grow up to 2 feet tall. The leaves grow directly on stems that come from the ground. These leaves are oval, dark green, and slightly wrinkled with fine hairs on them. They each have a deep vein down the middle, and the edges of the leaves are serrated. The flowers, which grow from the top of the stem, are small and purple with two lips arranged in rings around the stem. There are four stamens that come from each flower—two on the upper lip of the flower and two on the bottom lip. The seeds are very small, black, and irregular in size.

Parts used: Leaves

Cautions: None known

Folklore and history: There is a lot of medicinal lore written about wood betony. As far back as Augustus Caesar's time, it was seen as an herb that could cure anything and was written about as a form of medicine that could preserve the liver and help with digestion. In medieval medicine it was a panacea, including for the bites of venomous serpents and mad dogs. There is some lore about using wood betony to repel the fey as well.

Spiritual uses: Aiding rituals and protection from Witchcraft, serpents, dragons, and the fey

Spiritual anecdote: This is one of those underutilized herbs in herbal medicine and in magical practice. When I worked at an herb store in Minneapolis, there was a man that came in at least once a month, asking me for medicinal advice and herbs that would cure this or that. One day he asked me if I knew how to get rid of a dragon that was stalking him. Not missing a beat, I asked him if the dragon was a friend or if it wished him harm. The man said that he didn't know and didn't want to find out. After some more probing, I found out that he had pissed off a man who said he was a warlock and claimed to have possession of fire-breathing dragons. The story got weirder; the man said that he saw a small dragon out of the corner of his eye before he got into his car, and when he went to turn on his car, a big puff of smoke came from under the hood. That freaked him out a bit, but then he went home to find that his brand-new seven-day candle, which hadn't been lit yet, was burned down to the bottom. So, the next day that I was at the store after that, he came to me asking for help. I created a formula for him out of a few protective herbs, including wood betony, and mumbled a protection spell over the blend. I told him to carry it and burn it as incense while saying a prayer of his choice. He came back the following month and said that he hadn't seen the dragon for a few weeks and that no other fire-related issues had happened.

Astrological association: Juniper

Deities, angels, or spirit associations: Hercules, Demeter, and Athena

Meditation: *May fear or harm flee from me while betony stands beside me.*

Magical spell: This herb can be used for protection not only against animals or spirits but against people who behave snake- or mad-doglike as well. This is best accomplished by putting a little in a small bag with some other protective herbs and a protective charm.

Borage (*Borago officinalis*)

Common names: Herb of gladness and starflower

Description: Borage is an annual that is 1 to 1½ feet tall with bright blue, five-pointed flowers that droop in small clusters. In the center of the flower is a cone. The leaves are up to 5 inches long and ovate to basal in shape. They have a silvery-green appearance that is caused by silvery-white hairs on its leaves and stems. The flowers are edible and taste like cucumbers.

Parts used: Leaves, seeds, and flowers

Cautions: Use the leaf internally in small amounts due to its pyrrolizidine alkaloid content; according to current research, the seed oil and flower are safe to use. Do not use if pregnant, if breastfeeding, or if you have liver disease.

Folklore and history: Historically, borage was one of the herbs that was associated with happiness. Its bright and cheery nature made people merry and joyful. According to Dioscorides and Pliny, when it is steeped in wine, it brings absolute forgetfulness of problems. John Evelyn, a seventeenth-century diarist whose diary, *The Diary of John Evelyn*, was published after his death, wrote that borage was used "to revive the hypochondriac and cheer the hard student." Gerard, in *The Herbal*, recommended its use "to exhilarate and make the mind glad" and "drive away all sadnesse, dulnesse and melancholy" and said that "a syrup made of the flowers of Borage comforteth the heart, purgeth melancholy, and quieteth the phreneticke or lunaticke person."

Spiritual uses: Borage is well known as an herb of courage and an herb that increases psychic abilities, but by using observation and the doctrine of signatures, we can find a few other magical uses. The color and shape of the flowers, which grow in clusters that sway in the wind, tell me several things that have borne out with experimentation. Because of the blue flowers and the herb's medicinal actions, I can say that borage is a true healing plant that can calm the psyche and help with spells that involve healing both the mind and the body. It can also be used in spells to increase beauty and grace and be used to cool hot and uncomfortable situations. It can be burned in incense or crushed and put in shoes to increase courage. Borage can also be drunk as a tisane to promote natural grace and beauty.

Spiritual anecdote: One of my herbal clients came to see me once with her teenage daughter. Her daughter had an acne issue and was also distraught because she felt ugly and out of place at school. One of the spiritual treatments I gave to her was a packet of charmed and beauty-charged borage seeds. I told her and her mother to plant them in a place where they would be seen and tended to every day. I told the young lady that once the plants bloomed, she was to ingest one flower daily from the dark moon to the full moon and carry a flower with her daily to school. Two months after the flowers started blooming, the young lady was glowing with both inner and outer beauty and, at our follow-up appointment, told me she had met a young man to date.

Astrological association: Jupiter

Deities, angels, or spirit associations: Aphrodite, Brigid, and Diana

Meditation: *Herb of happiness, herb of light, help me heal and become beautiful and bright.*

Magical spell: To create inner beauty and happiness and bring joy into your life, grow borage in the spring. When the plant blooms, take one flower daily, from dark moon to full, and eat it while saying the plant's meditation.

Burdock (*Arctium lappa*)

Common names: Bardana, bardane, great burdock, great bur, hardock, hareburr, hurr-bur, turkey burrseed, cocklebur, beggar's buttons, cockle button, lappa, thorny burr, fox's clote, love leaves, personata, clotbur, and happy major

Description: Burdock is a large biennial plant that reaches up to 6 feet tall in its second year. Its root is large in width, starchy in the first year and hollow in the second year. The root extends into a long taproot, which can exceed 12 inches and have multiple rootlets. The leaves in the first year come out in a rosette pattern. They are smaller the first year of growth, varying from 6 to 12 inches in length and ovate, and in the second year, the leaves can get as big as 3 feet long and 1½ feet wide and are more ovate chordate. The leaves are a deep green on the top and gray underneath due to fine hairs and may have a reddish tinge to the stalk that supports them. In the plant's second year, it sends up a stalk with leaves that alternate, and in July flowers are borne in clusters at the top of the stem. The small, feathery flowers are purple and tubular in nature; they sit upon a globular-shaped base that is covered with stiff, hooked bracts.

Once the flower dies, the seed is enclosed in a spiked pod with hooked bracts that attach to everything that passes by. The seedpod is multicelled and has stiff, sharp white hairs. The seeds are dark brown to black and slightly oily.

Parts used: Leaves, seeds, and roots and rhizomes

Cautions: Diabetics should monitor blood sugars while taking any part of the plant internally. Do not use during pregnancy, if you have allergies to plants in the composite family (Asteraceae), or if you're taking insulin or oral antidiabetic agents. It may cause allergic dermatitis when collecting.

Folklore and history: Burdock is famous for its hooked burrs. Its botanical name comes from *arktos*, which is a Greek word that means "bear," suggesting rough-coated fruits, and *lappa*, which means "to seize." Culpeper wrote that it "wonderfully help the biting of any serpents, and helpeth those that are bit by a wild dog." It is said that burdock was the inspiration for the modern-day wonder called Velcro.

Spiritual uses: Healing, protection, and fertility; it can also be used to increase the power of a spell (think of the plant's determination). You can also cast the leaves around the house to ward off negativity and to aid in protection. The first-year root, harvested in the spring, can be eaten in a ritual dish to increase endurance or fertility for Beltane. When using burdock in incense, only use a small amount of leaves because they smell bitter when burned. A tincture made of the seeds taken daily can increase fertility and sexual endurance. You can carry the seedpods or burrs of the plant with you for protection on a daily basis, or you can let this plant grow along the edge of your land to protect your property. Root pieces can also be carried in pouches for healing, fertility, or protection.

Spiritual anecdote: I use burdock to assist in the protection of my property. The plants seem to spring up on the edges of my land and serve as guardians to protect the area within. They've protected me in other areas as well. One day, while harvesting herbs on the night of a full moon on a friend's land, I heard voices and movement from the forest (where people often hunted). I hunched down and asked the spirits of the plants to protect me, and as I did, I heard one of the voices start hurling expletives. It seemed they had walked into a burdock and nettle patch. I then heard the voices get farther away. Plants to the rescue again!

Astrological association: Saturn or Venus

Deities, angels, or spirit associations: Demeter and Loki

Meditation: Sticky, spiky, thorny one with leaves so large, protect me against my enemies, protect me from harm. Shield me from those who may hurt me; keep me safe within your protective arms.

Magical spell: For fertility, gather the first-year roots in the waning moon, cut them into small pieces, and carve symbols of fertility or prosperity in them; string the root beads on red thread and let them dry. Once they've dried, hang them over your bed for fertility.

Calendula (*Calendula officinalis*)

Common names: Pot marigold, marybud, marygold, gold-bloom, garden marigold, holigold, golds, ruddes, ruddles, mary gowles, spouse solis, and bride of the sun

Description: Calendula is an annual plant with angular, branched stems and prominent, pale green spatulate sessile leaves with widely spaced border teeth, which alternate along the stems and exude a sticky substance. The whole plant stands 1 to 2 feet tall. Its bright orange or yellow many-petaled flower rays are borne on a crown-shaped floret, and as the petals drop off, a circular corona of seeds remains. It looks like a miniature sun. The calendula plant reseeds easily in the garden from year to year. The parts often collected are the flower tops, and they should be collected in the morning, once the dew has dried, between the months of June and September.

Parts used: Dried flower heads and petals

Cautions: None known

Folklore and history: In the twelfth century, Macer wrote that merely looking at the plant would improve eyesight, clear the head, and encourage cheerfulness. Culpeper, in his book *Culpeper's Complete Herbal & English Physician*, recommended it to "strengthen the heart," and it was highly regarded in the treatment of smallpox and measles. Used historically as poor man's saffron, calendula adds both color and a saffron-like flavor to foods. Calendula's name is a reference to its tendency to bloom in accordance with the calendar.

Spiritual uses: Magically, calendula has many qualities that bear mentioning. It has the ability to cause visionary-type dreams, increase innate psychic abilities, and increase the amount of joy in life. Place a flower under your pillow and think of a question before you go to sleep, and in the morning, you should have an answer. The flower petals make a delicious psychic tisane; drink it daily to improve clairvoyance and divination skills. Integrate this herb into your daily routine to produce happiness and joy in both your magical and your mundane life. Calendula is also a favorite flower of the fey. If you plant it in your garden, you may be able to see one of these magical creatures hiding in the petals.

Spiritual anecdote: I had an herbal client who was devastated; her dog had died six months earlier. I could sympathize because my animals are my children, but her depression was affecting her job. Her doctor had prescribed antidepressants, but these made her feel sluggish and even more despondent. I had her drink an herbal tea of lemon balm, hibiscus, borage flowers, and calendula while meditating on how much she loved her dog and that even if he was not there physically, he would always be next to her as an angel. She felt an immediate lifting of the sadness, and over the next week, she got progressively happier and more clearheaded. She stopped the antidepressants, and within the next three months, she got a new puppy.

Astrological association: Sun

Deities, angels, or spirit associations: Apollo, Brigid, Isis, Lugh, and Cerridwen

Meditation: Concentrate on the bright petals of the flower and say: *May your bright sunshine light the way toward seeing the truth in all things; may your rays of sunshine clear the cloudiest sky.*

Magical spell: To help improve psychic ability, make a cup of tea, adding 1 part calendula, 1 part mugwort, and 1 part vervain. Steep it for at least thirteen minutes, and then recite the plant's meditation while concentrating on your goal.

Catnip (*Nepeta cataria*)

Common names: Catnep, catrup, catswort, cataria, and field balm

Description: Catnip is an erect shrub-like herb that grows up to 1 foot tall. The ovate leaves are 1 to 1½ inches long, soft, whitish green, and serrated with hairy undersides. The flowers are white to pale blue and lipped with crimson dots on the edges; they are arranged in small tight whorls with long sepals. The plant's musky mint odor is distinctive and emitted when touched. Catnip is a common plant that grows wild in many places. It is said to be a perennial but only lives for about two to three years; it reseeds, however, and an ample supply can be easily found. One of the funniest signatures of this plant is its ability to intoxicate cats. It makes them frisky and playful due to the musk-like pheromones it exudes.

Parts used: Leaves and flowering tops

Cautions: Do not use while pregnant or concurrently with echinacea or prescription sedatives, as it may intensify their effect.

Folklore and history: In *Culpeper's Complete Herbal & English Physician*, he writes that "the juice drunk in wine is good for bruises." The leaves, when smoked, give a mild euphoria that's similar to cannabis.

Spiritual uses: This herb is a spiritual person's dream. It helps prepare you for meditation or journey work by making tensions of the mundane world dissolve, allowing you to slip into a meditative state. I have also used this herb in love, money, and healing magic. For love magic I usually mix it with rose petals, lavender, or orange flowers and recommend burning it as incense or drinking it as an herbal tea. In hoodoo if a woman carries catnip in a flannel bag, men will be attracted to her. Another hoodoo ritual is to sprinkle a catnip tisane at the four corners of the bed to attract a new lover. Catnip is also known to attract luck to the person who finds or grows it; I often carry a leaf of it on me when I am in need of some extra luck or money.

Spiritual anecdote: I once used this herb to help a woman feel more beautiful. She was already good looking, but she had low self-esteem and thought she was ugly, and it was affecting her relationships. I had her drink a cup of catnip tea every evening while meditating on a beautiful picture of Venus as she repeated the following three times: "I am as beautiful as the sunrise in the morning and as powerful as the ocean as it meets the shore." It took her only a week before she had dreams of Venus, who gave her visions and gifts. Within a month she said she felt as beautiful as nature itself and was feeling like asking a man at work on a date.

Astrological association: Venus

Deities, angels, or spirit associations: Bast, Sekhmet, Freya, and Aphrodite

Meditation: Prior to journey work, drink a cup of catnip tea, then imagine a doorway. There is a curtain covering the opening so you cannot see what's on the other side. Walk through it. In front of you is another doorway with a curtain covering the opening, but this time the curtain is thinner, and you can see something beyond. You walk through it. You see a third doorway, and there is, again, a curtain, but it is almost sheer. Walk through it and you will be at the start of your journey.

Magical spell: For a love spell, mix equal parts rose petals, catnip, and lavender together. While blending it, concentrate on your intentions. Once the mix is ready, you can either burn it as incense or carry it around with you.

Cedar (*Thuja occidentalis*)

Common names: Arborvitae, tree of life, white cedar, yellow cedar, American cedar, and hackmatack

Description: Cedar is an evergreen conifer that can reach a height of 20 feet. The branches are short, and the lower ones are horizontal, while the upper ones crown to form a dense, conical head. The leaves grow on short stems in opposite pairs. They are bright green in color and resemble overlapping scales. The leaves have an aromatic odor when crushed. The small, solitary terminal flowers appear from April to July and are yellowish green. The cone is small and pale green when young; it's a light, reddish brown with thin scales when mature.

Parts used: Young twigs and leaves

Cautions: It should not be taken during pregnancy or lactation; cedar should be avoided internally due to its toxic nature.

Folklore and history: Many Native American tribes have stories about this herb. Most of the tribal folklore that I have heard refer to it as a tree of purification and communication with the ancestors. In fact, it is sometimes used in sweat lodges as a purification herb on the rocks. The smoke is sacred and not only purifies the spirit but sends the prayers and songs of the people to their ancestors and gods. According to Native American lore, it is also used for heart pain or sadness. In European lore the tree was associated with death. When a limb fell off a tree near a house, it signified the death of a family member.

Spiritual uses: Purification, relief of sadness or heartache, sending messages to the gods, and healing; when hung in the home, it can protect against lightning. It can also be an omen of upcoming death.

Spiritual anecdote: I remember going to a Native American ceremony and sweat once where cedar was used to purify a woman who had been burdened by the death of several family members. The shaman and medicine woman thought the family had been cursed because of a family member's unjust act toward an elder. The woman was cleansed with smoke before the ceremony with white sage and then cedar. During the sweat, cedar was put on the rocks at almost every round. After the ceremony, the woman, who was barely able to stand, was taken from the sweat and again cleaned with cedar and then with sweet grass (to bring the good spirits to help her). The woman recovered and had no further issues with bad luck or family deaths.

Astrological association: Sun

Deities, angels, or spirit associations: White Buffalo Calf Woman, Hecate, and Woden

Meditation: Cedar, please in thy infinite wisdom protect me from harm and allow healing to take place; free me from the influences that are causing me harm.

Magical spells: A piece taken and put in a bag to be worn will protect the wearer from harm and lightning. Burning the plant as incense will clean the air of harmful or negative influences and will keep negative forces away for a period of time.

Celery (*Apium graveolens*)

Common names: Celery fruit, celery seed, smallage, and wild celery

Description: Celery is a strong-smelling, erect biennial plant that grows up to 24 inches tall. The stalks are bright green, ribbed, and stringy. Celery has bright green leaves that are pinnate with large, toothed leaflets whose footstalks alternate up the main stem. The flowers are small, white, and contain five double petals. These flowers grow in four to ten simple umbels, which come together under a semiglobular umbel. The seeds are small, light brown, and compressed, forming ridges along the lateral border.

Parts used: Dried ripe seeds and aerial parts

Caution: Don't ingest during pregnancy and lactation.

Folklore and history: Ancient documents show that celery has been cultivated for at least three thousand years, notably in Pharaonic Egypt. It was known in China in 450 BC, and around that same time, the ancient Greeks on the Isthmus of Corinth regularly awarded their winning athletes with crowns of celery stems and leaves. They also used celery to make wine to serve as a reward in the athletic games. To help get rid of dizziness, witches were thought to eat the seeds of the plant before flying off on their besoms. Medicinal preparations began to emerge in the late nineteenth century, and these generally contained the juice of crushed celery seeds.

Spiritual uses: Psychic development and sexuality spells

Spiritual anecdote: I use celery seed and celery as an aphrodisiac on a regular basis, and my favorite case involving celery was a client who had a husband who preferred watching football to lovemaking. My client made his favorite hot wings and celery with ranch dressing, and while making the ranch dressing from a packet and cutting the celery, she chanted, "Lover, come to me; let this celery remind you of your other passions." She gave the celery and ranch dressing to him during the game and then sprinkled celery seed from the living room to the bed where she had hot wings and celery waiting for him. When he got there, she fed him some celery, and needless to say, he forgot about his game.

Astrological association: Mercury

Deities, angels, or spirit associations: Hermes and Aphrodite

Meditation: As an aphrodisiac, say: *Love, come to me as many times as seeds do I have; love, come to me in abundance now!*

Magical spells: Carry the seeds to attract sexual partners. You can also drink a tisane containing mugwort, celery seed, and wild lettuce to enhance psychic ability.

Chamomile (*Matricaria chamomilla*)

Common names: Momile, Roman chamomile, English chamomile, German chamomile, and wild chamomile

Description: Chamomile is an annual but freely reseeds itself yearly and is one of the few plants that thrives and spreads when stepped on. It rarely grows more than 1 foot tall, no matter the individual species. The semi globular center of the flower is about ¾ inch wide and bright yellow, and its petals are white and radiate out from the center. It has feathery leaves that are approximately 3 to 4 inches long. The flower has a sweet, apple-honey-like smell, and the ovate seeds are flat and numerous.

Parts used: Flowers

Cautions: Do not use if allergic to plants in the composite family (Asteraceae).

Folklore and history: In medieval times chamomile was one of the herbs strewn on the floors of homes because people thought the herb would chase away the plague. Chamomile has also been used for centuries in love spells. Victorian women would drink an herbal blend containing this herb before bed in hopes of seeing who their true love would be while they slept.

Spiritual uses: Preventing the plague, relief from depression, and attracting love, money, and protection; Chamomile tea can be sprinkled around the parameter of a house to both protect the inhabitant from harm and to attract money.

Spiritual anecdote: My teacher Matthew Wood taught me that chamomile is good for the two-year-old of any age (meaning that it is good for people who throw temper tantrums), but I never thought of using it in that way until a case presented itself to me. I was seeing a woman who said that her husband had changed after a car accident. He had gotten a concussion and experienced no other physical issues except for a stiff neck, but ever since the accident, he became angry over little things and resorted to throwing adult temper tantrums when he did not get his way. I had my client add some chamomile tea to his daily food, and he started calming down. As part of her spiritual treatment, I had her cleanse her house, and as she was using an herbal wand, she saw a thin black smoke leave her husband. It's possible that the angriness was coming from an opportunistic spirit who had possessed him, and between the herbal tea and the cleansing, it figured out it wasn't welcome. He was much nicer after the cleansing and the tea.

Astrological association: Sun

Deities, angels, or spirit associations: Apollo, Athena, Zeus, and Hera

Meditation: Mother of all the plants, please guide me on my journey, grant me peace, and (insert your wish for money, love, or protection here).

Magical spell: To attract love, make chamomile tea, put it in a spray bottle, and spray it on your face and clothes before leaving the house while saying, "Sunny flower, help me to shine as you do and help attract my true love to me."

Cinnamon (*Cinnamomum zeylanicum*)

Common names: Ceylon cinnamon, true cinnamon, and kwai

Description: The cinnamon tree grows up to 50 feet tall in subtropical to tropical regions. The outer bark is a smooth gray and has irregularly-sized, white dots growing on it. The inner bark is brownish red in color and is harvested from the tree. The harvested bark is known as a quill. The oval leaves come off the branches in an irregular pattern, and they are glossy and dark green with deep yellow-green veins. The flowers are small and pale yellow with five petals; they grow in racemes at the end of the branches. The berries produced from the flowers are purple, and each fruit has one black seed. All parts of the tree have the familiar cinnamon smell.

Parts used: Inner bark

Cautions: Cinnamon can lower the blood sugar when large amounts are eaten. The essential oil can burn when used on the skin, inhaled, or ingested.

Folklore and history: In medieval Europe, around AD 1300, cinnamon was more valuable than gold, and kings and empires fought over who would own the rights to trade or sell the spice. These battles only ended because it was found that the tree could be grown and farmed in other regions. Cinnamon was one of the herbs used in the mummification process, and it was burned as incense in Egyptian, Indian, and Chinese temples.

Spiritual uses: Purification, consecration of tools, love, lust, protection, and money

Spiritual anecdote: I had a friend who asked me, "How do I make someone fall in love with me?" After I had the it-is-important-not-to-work-that-kind-of-magic conversation with her, we discussed simple ways to make her more attractive and the belief that the best way to win a man's love is through his stomach. It's an old saying, but there is some truth and magic behind it. If you prepare a meal for someone, they automatically feel loved, and if you happen to put some herbs in there that are tasty and serve a magical purpose, it's a win-win situation. She found out the man she had a crush on loved cinnamon rolls, so I told her to make some for him and see what happened. Well, of course he loved her baking, and after three weeks of her baking for him, he started to like her. As for her, she was so tired of baking just to get this man to notice her that she got over her infatuation quite quickly and moved on to someone who didn't require as much work.

Astrological association: Sun

Deities, angels, or spirit associations: Sekhmet, Vishnu, and Lakshmi

Meditation: For safety and the ability to persevere, say: *Cinnamon, grant me the protection and strength to get through* (insert need).

Magical spell: Mix equal parts cinnamon, frankincense, and basil and burn while imagining you already have the money or prosperity that you need. Carry a small amount of the incense blend in your purse or wallet.

Cinquefoil, Creeping (*Potentilla reptans*)

Common names: Five-finger grass, crampweed, tormentil, and potentilla

Description: Cinquefoil has a low-creeping habit. The roots are blackish in color and thick near the base of the plant. The roots branch out via thin, delicate runners deep in the soil. The leaves come directly off the dark stem in a rosette pattern, growing alternatively up the stem. The leaves are compound, meaning that they have five or more distinct leaflets, which is where the plant gets the name five-finger grass from. The leaves are oval shaped with deeply serrated edges. They are dark green on the top and a lighter green on the bottom due to the short, fine hairs on the bottom of each leaf. The flowers are medium-sized and bright yellow with five petals. Each petal is double lobed, giving the appearance of ten petals.

Parts used: Leaves and roots

Cautions: None known

Folklore and history: Cinquefoil is one of those herbs that has historically been used more as a magical plant than a medicinal one, and it has a strong association with witches using it in spells. Traditionally, cinquefoil was mostly used for love magic but, according to M. Grieve, has also been used to make a bait for fish that guaranteed a heavy haul. As Grieve writes in *A Modern Herbal*, it was also used in a recipe for flying ointment, which, in addition to cinquefoil, included wolfsbane, smallage, and the fat of a baby who had been dug up from their grave. In addition to love spells and flying ointment, cinquefoil has also been used to attract money. In hoodoo, its five leaves represent the hand, and it is used to repel evil and bring good luck. The Natchez gave it to people who were believed to be under a spell or bewitched.

Spiritual uses: Love, money, spell strengthening, and fishing magic

Spiritual anecdote: I love to make some of the formulas I find in my collection of herbal books, and when I saw a recipe for catching more fish in *A Modern Herbal,* I had to try it. I made the recipe, which called for boiling corn with marjoram, thyme, nettles, cinquefoil, and a leek, and took the magic-infused corn with me to catch walleyes in one of my favorite fishing lakes in Minnesota. I used my corn as bait, and the men fishing nearby used worms. I quietly chanted to the fish (here, fishy, fishy, come to me) to attract them to the bait, and to the men's amazement, I caught twice as many fish as they did. I have also used this herb to strengthen other spells, especially those involving love or money.

Astrological association: Jupiter

Deities, angels, or spirit associations: Hecate, Diana, and Aradia

Meditation: To attract money, say: *Plant of the witches, bring to me the money I need to thrive three times.*

Magical spell: To attract money, put cinquefoil in a red flannel or velvet bag, say the plant's meditation, sprinkle two drops of van van oil on the bag, and wear it every day. Refresh the oil daily.

Copal (*Protium copal*)

Common names: Copal and Aztec gold

Description: The copal tree can be found in the tropical parts of Mexico and Central America under the canopies of larger trees and grows to be approximately 98 feet tall. The leaves are dark green and have yellowish-green veins; they are long, lance shaped, and grow equally up the stem. The five-petaled flowers are small, whitish yellow, and grow in panicles at the end of the stem. The fruit is small and light brown with a small pit inside. The bark of the tree is grayish brown and has a rough appearance. The resin is harvested by making small cuts in the tree.

Parts used: Resin

Cautions: Copal is safe to use in small doses; it is all right to chew but should not be swallowed.

Folklore and history: Most of the lore about this plant comes from the Aztecs, and some of that lore is based off the ritual items found in their tombs. Some of the items found below the Great Temple in Tenochtit-lan included a box with copal-handled, sacred tools and figurines with cores of copal covered in a clay, stucco-type material and dressed in sacred costumes. These figures are believed to be sacred representations of Aztec deities who were placed at the base of the temple for protection. Aztecs used copal for incense, and it was also used in everyday life as a fixative in makeup, as a color fixative in masks, as chewing gum, and in dentistry to hold gems in individual teeth.

Spiritual uses: Purification, fertility, creativity, and shape-shifting

Spiritual anecdote: I once had an herbal client who was a painter who had lost her ability to create. She also had some health issues, so while we worked on those, I asked her if she burned candles or incense while she tried to paint. She did not. Since she had said she had Aztec blood, I recommended burning a stick of copal incense and an orange candle and asking for assistance from the great spirit to guide her in creating art. My client said it took a few times with this new routine, but after she got used to it, she started producing some of her best work.

Astrological association: Sun

Deities, angels, or spirit associations: Tonatiuh, Chalchiuhtlicue, and Chicomecóatl

Meditation: To inspire creativity, say: *Ancient spirit of the trees, purify me and set me free from my boundaries.*

Magical spell: Before starting any shape-shifting magic, burn some copal on a charcoal, and start chanting in a low voice, "Goddess of magic, who could turn herself into a lion, tiger, or anything, guide my journey to turn into the (insert what you want to change into)." As the incense continues to burn, start moving like the animal you want to shape-shift into and speak as this animal would. Keep a piece of copal in your clothes or in your hand as you start shape-shifting.

Cowslip (*Primula veris*)

Common names: Peagles, fairy cup, keywort, key flower, Peter's flower, key of heaven, and herba paralysis

Description: A perennial that is naturalized all over Europe but grows in temperate regions in Switzerland and North America, cowslip grows up to 10 inches tall, and its bright green leaves, which grow in a rosette pattern at the base of the plant, have deep veins down the centers. The edges of each leaf curl under a little. The plant has multiple thin green stems that pop up from the base of the plant, and each stem produces ten to thirty individual bright yellow blooms. The flower sepals are connected to form what looks like a small bladder at the base, which is where the flowers open from. Each flower has five petals about ½ inch wide. Some petals are a darker yellow or have a red dot near the area that connects to the base. The seeds are small and spread easily; the plant also spreads by underground runners.

Parts used: Leaves and flowers

Cautions: None known

Folklore and history: Cowslip has been referred to by many writers, from Pliny the Elder to Hildegard of Bingen, who discussed its powers. According to M. Grieve in *A Modern Herbal*, the cowslip flower was associated with Freya, "the key virgin," but researchers have argued that the association was probably with Hecate, as she was the virgin who held the keys to the afterlife. When Christianity came to Europe, many people started associating cowslip flowers with the Virgin Mary instead of Pagan goddesses.

Spiritual uses: Glamor magic, fey magic, underworld magic, and trance work; I love using cowslip to help people who have a hard time getting into a trance state. It is a mild hypnotic, and it helps to strengthen other herbs it's blended with. My favorite combination is cowslip flowers with vervain; I make a tincture with this combination to help people whose minds keep having mundane thoughts that keep them from meditating or doing trance work. I usually give ten to twenty drops depending on the need.

Spiritual anecdote: I once had a student who was a computer programmer who could not get code writing out of his head and relax enough to do meditation or trance work. We tried several herbs to help him, but then I remembered that he always lost his keys. Keys are associated with cowslip flowers in mythology, so we decided to try the herb. Not only was my client able to stop the codes he was programming from running through his head and relax enough to go into a deep trance state, but he told me that he didn't lose his keys for two weeks after he had the formula. He decided to use the combination at least once a week before he did a tarot reading and to keep him from losing his keys.

Astrological association: Sun

Deities, angels, or spirit associations: Diana and Hecate

Meditation: Beautiful flower, make me look beautiful, wise, and shine as you do.

Magical spell: For glamor magic, take a fresh cowslip flower and dry it well. Put it in a light blue flannel or felt bag and chant the flower's meditation as you concentrate on what glamor magic you want to happen. Carry the flower with you around your neck, tucked under your clothes. Be aware that glamor magic does not last long; the flower can lose power in just a few hours. Use sparingly.

Daisy *(Bellis perennis)*

Common names: Bruisewort, eyes, field daisy, common daisy, and moon daisy

Description: This perennial plant, also known as the common daisy, is often seen growing in people's yards and in areas disturbed by people throughout North America and Europe. The daisy grows about 6 to 12 inches tall with leaves that are long, lance shaped, and serrated that grow from a rosette. Multiple flowers grow from individual stalks coming from the rosettes. Each flower has a bright yellow disk at the center with between thirty-eight and forty-two white petals coming from it.

Parts used: Flowers

Cautions: None known

Folklore and history: Throughout history daisies were often associated with love and divination. According to M. Grieve, the chant "He loves me, he loves me not" goes back at least to the 1500s. Often young women would say this chant as they plucked off one petal at a time to determine whether their love was reciprocated.

Spiritual uses: The daisy has a lot to offer as an herb of love and pleasure. You can make an oil infused with daisies and add your favorite essential oil or wear daisies to attract love. It is also an herb of happiness and peace. Give a handful of magically charged daisies to bestow joy and peace to a person in need, or wear a chain of daisies to a summer ritual to honor the goddess. The magic this plant creates is powerful in its simplicity.

Fairies are also attracted to this flower; use them as flowers on your fairy altar or as an offering to the Queen of the Fairies. You may come back the next day to see the flowers woven into a beautiful daisy chain.

Spiritual anecdote: This herb can be used at midsummer to make wreaths for women's hair for ritual. Symbolically the flower by itself represents the sun or the god. Woven into a circle, the flowers represent the goddess. The weaving also symbolizes the love shared between the god and goddess. I used to do this in Minnesota at Beltane festivals with the women in my group. We wove them together while chanting, and later the women would hang them on their beds to promote love and peace or hang them near their fairy alters to attract the fey.

Astrological association: Sun or moon

Deities, angels, or spirit associations: Freya, Artemis, Thor, Belinus, Ra, and fairies, including the Queen of the Fairies

Meditation: As the sun shines on me, may the love of the goddess grow and strengthen me.

Magical spell: Gather 2 cups of fresh daisy heads and add them to 2 cups of oil in a jar. Seal the jar and let it sit in the sun from full moon to full moon. Once a moon cycle has passed, strain out the flowers and add your favorite essential oil to it (lavender, rose, and rose geranium are all good scents). Wear the oil to attract love, happiness, or inner peace.

Dandelion (*Taraxacum officinale*)

Common names: Lion's-tooth, fairy clock, blowball, *pissenlit*, pee-the-bed, cankerwort, priest's-crown, puffball, swine snout, white endive, and wild endive

Description: This plant grows up to 24 inches tall and starts out as a rosette of characteristic lion's-tooth leaves that can be up to 14 inches long. The leaves are lance shaped with deep indentations, or teeth, along the borders. The flower stems, which are slightly hairy, grow directly from the base of the rosette and bear yellow flower heads made up of 100 or more bisexual florets. These give way to the familiar puffball of greenish-brown seeds that have silky threads arranged in a globe pattern, which allows them to be easily caught by the wind. The long taproot rises from a short rhizome. The root is covered with a thin, dark brown bark but is whitish yellow inside. The roots, like the stems and leaves, produce a bitter-tasting, white, milky sap that is sticky.

Parts used: Leaves, flowers, and roots

Cautions: Do not take dandelion internally if there is an occlusion of the bile ducts or gallbladder empyema.

Folklore and history: The ancient Greeks wore crowns of dandelions to worship the goddess Venus, and dandelions are known to be a favorite of the fairy folk. Some say that if you go out on a moonlit night and open a closed dandelion head, you may find a fairy hiding inside, and then it must grant you a wish.

Dandelion was first mentioned in Chinese herbals as early as the seventh century, and in Europe it first appears in the *Ortus Sanitatis* by Jacob Meydenbach. It was used by the Arabian physicians of the tenth and eleventh centuries for its diuretic properties. Dandelion's common name was apparently invented by Master Wilhelm, a fifteenth-century surgeon who compared the shape of the leaves to the shape of a lion's tooth. There is a lot of British lore about it being bad luck for children to pick dandelion because it makes them wet the bed. In folklore one of the old uses for the puffball seed head was telling time. A person would blow on it three times, and however many tufts were left was what time it was.

Dandelions grow in all parts of the world, and the seeds were brought to America by settlers so that they could have a reliable spring green to eat. The leaves may be used as a salad vegetable in spring before it flowers, the roasted root can be used as a coffee substitute, and the flowers can be used to make wine.

Spiritual uses: Purification, divination, strength, wishes, and fertility; an infusion or infused oil of the root will promote physic powers. I make this oil and keep it on hand to anoint the third eye before doing psychic workings. A cup of dandelion tea placed steaming at the front door or bedside will call spirits. The flowers, when in their puffball state, have many spiritual uses. In order to find out what time it is, blow on the mature seed head three times; the number of seeds left is the time. In order to find out how long you will live, blow on the seed head once and count the remaining seeds. To send a message to a loved one, blow the seed head in their direction. If all of the seeds are blown off with one breath, your loved one will return your message. In order to make a wish come true, blow all the seeds off with one breath. To make a wish with the flower, whisper your wish to the plant, and toss it over your left shoulder into a stream of running water; don't look back or the wish will not come true. I have made wishes using this method with good results.

Spiritual anecdote: One of my favorite case studies with this plant involved a woman who had issues trying to see fairies. She had a beautiful fairy altar with little houses and pathways, and she just wanted to see one. We talked about offerings that may appeal to them (honey and jelly beans) and how to sneak up on them and perhaps catch a glimpse. I told her to leave offerings in the dandelion field near her house and to watch the dandelions open up as the sun came out. She managed to see a small, bright green light with wings come out of one of the dandelions as it was opening. She was so happy because she finally saw a fairy.

Astrological associations: Sun and Jupiter

Deities, angels, or spirit associations: Hecate, Zeus, Apollo, Sekhmet, Aphrodite, Hermes, and the Queen of the Fairies

Meditation: *Flower of the sun, shine upon me brightly and grant me my deepest desire. Open the door; show me the way to my destiny.*

Magical spells: To attract fairies, put this flower on your indoor fairy altar. If your altar is outside, spread some seeds from a dandelion puffball around the altar and let them grow. If you want to see fairies sleeping inside the closed flower buds, leave out a glass of mead or sweet wine in a bed of dandelions. Get up before dawn and tiptoe to the area where you left the mead or wine. If the glass is empty, you may have some fairies sleeping nearby; carefully peel back the petals of a dandelion near the mead, and see if there's a fairy inside. You may be surprised by what you see. Fairies can disguise themselves as brightly colored insects or bright lights if they are caught sleeping.

Dragon's Blood (*Calamus draco*)

Common names: Blood, blume, dragon's blood palm, and dove's blood

Description: Calamus draco, the source of dragon's blood resin, is a small palm tree that grows in subtropical regions but is mostly collected and shipped from the Canary Islands. It can grow up to 50 feet tall, and its trunk grows straight with the branches growing from the top of the trunk instead of along the whole trunk. The bark is light gray in color and smooth to the touch. The leaves grow alternately up stems that extend from the ends of each branch. The leaves are a yellow-green color and grow up to 2 feet long in a fanlike shape. The flowers are small, white, and grow along small panicles off the tips of the branches. From each flower comes an oval, brownish-red fruit that is about 1 inch long. Each berry has scales that look like a dragon's scales and is covered with a sticky resin. This resin is harvested and sold as dragon's blood.

The export of dragon's blood is heavily regulated, and this can make this resin more costly than some of the others. The resin itself comes not from the sap of the tree but from the coating on the outside of the tree's berries. Traditionally, the berries are put in a bag and rubbed vigorously until heat forms, which allows the resinous coating to be released. This substance is then collected and rolled in palm leaves before being stored in a drying hut. After the resin has dried, the leaves are removed and the resin is formed into teardrop-shaped drupes, which are then sold with a gold seal on them. Drupes are later broken into chunks by merchants so they can be sold by weight.

Parts used: Resin

Cautions: None known

Folklore and history: On the Canary Islands, this resin is used for a variety of medicinal uses. There is some lore on it being used for purification in incense and by sprinkling the powder around the doors.

Spiritual uses: Protection, love, lust, purification, and strengthening spells; I have found dragon's blood resin to work well as an aphrodisiac when mixed with jasmine and roses and burned as incense. Dragon's blood oil can be substituted for real blood when concocting a nonedible brew or writing spells. Dragon's blood has no smell of its own, so it can be scented in whatever way you want.

Spiritual anecdote: I use this resin in so many ways to improve the strength of my spells. Usually, adding a small amount to magical blends is enough to amplify a spell. I also use it as a substitute for blood in recipes and to write with. I anoint my magical tools with it after I clean them, and the resin helps seal the wood and metal against the salt, water, and candle wax that eventually always seems to get on altar tools. The resin also helps keep the power in the tools, building up their strength over time.

Astrological association: Mars

Deities, angels, or spirit associations: Oshun, Yemaja, and Persephone

Meditation: Draco the dragon, ruler of the night skies, grant me my wish, push it toward the heavens, and let your fiery breath intensify its abilities.

Magical spell: To make infused oil of dragon's blood, gather 1 cup of dragon's blood resin chunks and 2 cups of a carrier oil (this can be almond, olive, or whatever you have handy). Add the oil to a saucepan, then add the dragon's blood resin. Turn your stove on to the lowest setting and melt the resin in the oil. This process requires a lot of stirring so the resin doesn't burn to the bottom of the pan. You should make this oil in a double boiler if you have access to one.

Echinacea (*Echinacea purpurea*)

Common names: Purple coneflower, black sampson, Kansas snakeroot, rudbeckia, American narrow-leaved coneflower, and spider flower

Description: Echinacea is a perennial herb, up to 2 feet tall, with simple, rough stems that are hollow near the base and thicken slightly close to the flower head. The leaves are elongated, slightly elliptical with entire margins that are covered with coarse hairs. The defining feature of the flower is its centrally located cone, which is surrounded by rough, hairy bracts and down-turned, light purple ray florets. The branched and tapered root is grayish brown and flecked with white.

Parts used: Whole plant, especially the roots and rhizomes

Cautions: Do not overuse this herb because it is currently being overharvested and is at risk for extinction.

Folklore and history: Echinacea is one of those herbs that almost everyone has heard of, but what do you really know about it? *Echinacea purpurea* is prairie native, and it has been used for hundreds of years by Indigenous peoples to cure snake bites and all kinds of serious infections. There weren't a lot of magical associations written about it, except to say it was protective and healing in nature.

Spiritual uses: As mentioned in the folklore and history section, not much has been written about the use of echinacea, but by observing the plant, we can think of some very appropriate uses. One of the most prominent features of the echinacea plant is its cone head. This is actually the seed head; it is tipped in a black color and stiff to the touch. The plant reseeds easily, so new volunteer plants appear early in the spring, often several feet around the original. These signatures indicate that echinacea could be used for determination, strength, healing, and fertility. If you are planning on getting pregnant or need inner strength, you should carry some seeds with you in a bag or put them under your pillow at night. Its use as an aphrodisiac and fertility herb will be helpful, especially if an infection, such as syphilis, or some other venereal disease was involved in reducing fertility. Echinacea also contains a spiritual energy that is pure grace and knowledge; I would use it magically to not only give inner strength but to give inner wisdom.

Spiritual anecdote: I knew a Dakota shaman who used this herb to draw poison—not snake venom but societal poison—out of people. Once I saw him use the plant, dirt and all, on a member of his tribe who had an issue with alcohol. This was not a normal alcohol addiction but a rabid addiction. This man would guzzle brandy until he passed out; twice he almost died from alcohol poisoning. He told the shaman that he couldn't help himself; it was like he was possessed by the Devil in the alcohol, and he had to drink it until it was coming out of his pores. The man said that he didn't want to drink anymore because it had caused him to lose everything. The shaman put the whole plant on the man's solar plexus area, shook the plant, and asked it to take out the evil spirit that was causing him to drink. The man did stop drinking for a while after that, and while he did return to drinking, he did not drink as much and was able to control it better.

Astrological association: Jupiter

Deities, angels, or spirit associations: Raphael, Hermes, and Hecate

Meditation: Herb of protection, assist me to protect me and aid me in my time of need.

Magical spells: Carry some of the roots in a bag for personal protection, or grow it in your garden to protect the surrounding property from harm. It can also be used as an aphrodisiac when trying to conceive a child.

Elder (*Sambucus nigra*)

Common names: Sambucus, European elder, black elder, black-berried elder, pipe tree, common elder, bore tree, boor tree, bourtree, bountry, ellanwood, ellhorn, German elder, and *ueldrum*

Description: Elderberry is a shrubby tree that grows up to 12 feet in height with a width of 6 feet. The bark is light gray when young and changes to a darker gray with long, narrow furrows that develop with age. The stems of the elderberry bush are pithy and hollow, which allows them to bend easily. The leaves grow up to 12 inches long and grow opposite of each other. They have an odd number of compound pinnate leaves with two or three pairs of lateral leaflets that are lance shaped and coarsely toothed. The bisexual flowers are small, yellowish white in color, and appear in early summer; they are arranged in large, flat clusters. The saucer-shaped flowers have a short, bell-shaped calyx and five stamens. Berries are attached to the flat cluster by a short, green stem. The berry itself is initially green and matures to a dark purple. It has several small, dark brown seeds within the fruit.

Parts used: Dried flowers, berries, inner bark, and leaves

Caution: The bark should not be used in pregnancy, as it is a strong purgative, while the unripe berries, young bark, and leaves contain the toxic glycoside D-sambunigrin, which can produce hydrocyanic acid.

Folklore and history: Elder wood has long been associated with sorrow and death; baby cradles made from the wood were said to kill the child in it or attract the fey to exchange a changeling for the infant. In M. Grieve's *A Modern Herbal*, she states that the wood of an elder tree was what Christ's crucifixion cross was made of and that it was from an elder tree that Judas hanged himself. Throughout Europe, especially amongst the Romani people, it was widely believed that burning elder wood brought bad luck, and great care was taken to avoid burning it. In contrast, there is also the historical use of hanging elder branches in the house to provide protection against lightning strikes, witches, and negative magic.

In Germany Frau Holda, a dryad called Hyldemoer in England, is the guardian spirit of this tree. Be careful during harvest of the fresh berries or in cutting an elder down or the spirit will come out and curse you. In fact, there is a special way to harvest it to avoid bad luck. First you should make an offering to the bush and tell Frau Holda what you plan to do with the plant, then ask her permission to harvest from the plant, making sure to be very respectful. Traditionally, this is done with a bowed head (no hat on the head) and the arms together, as if in prayer. Once a period of silence has passed, you may hear her approval. If she gives you permission, first make a small cut in the wood to allow the spirit to escape, and then harvest your berries or wood. Once you are done, thank Frau Holda and back away respectfully.

It is said that the pith of elder was hollowed out and flutes were made from the stems, which could be used to call the fey. In Denmark the lore is that if you stand under an elder bush on Midsummer Eve at midnight, you would see the King of the Fairies ride by in his chariot. Historically, it was used in treating the bites of sea serpents or mad dogs, which caused madness.

Spiritual uses: Protection against lightning strikes, thieves, and negative Witchcraft; it should be noted that, according to legend, if you mistreat the plant you could be struck by lightning or have a period of bad luck. It is a tree to be respected and honored. If you rescue elder from destruction or help spread seeds in the fall, the spirit of the bush will assist you in your magical needs. Flutes can be made from its hollowed-out stems to call the fairies, and the plant can also be used to help in cases of madness.

Spiritual anecdotes: I use elder in my home to protect it against thieves; I have branches in each window and over each door. Elder has a special place in my heart, and I use it for everything, from making cough syrup to fairy furniture. I have rescued many elder bushes, often transplanting them from mowed areas to safe areas in the woods, along stream banks, or in my yard.

Astrological association: Venus

Deities, angels, or spirit associations: Hecate, the Morrigan, Faru Holda, Aphrodite, Persephone, and Demeter

Meditation: Dear mother plant, grant me the wisdom to honor you and show me how to use your secrets for the good of all.

Magical spells: For protection against thieves, take two pieces of elder wood and tie them together with red thread. Carry this with you or put it somewhere you have valuables you want to protect. To chase negativity from a household and reverse the evil eye, burn elder leaves on a charcoal and walk sunwise around the home.

Elecampane (*Inula helenium*)

Common names: Helenium grandiflorum, Aster officinalis, Aster helenium, Alant, elfwort, elf dock, velvet dock, scabwort, yellow starwort, wild sunflower, elecampagne, horseheal, and horse elder

Description: Elecampane can grow up to 6 feet tall and 3 feet wide. It has a thick, cylindrical rhizome that spreads through the earth and an erect, tough, deeply furrowed stem that has fine hairs at the top and thicker ones at the bottom. The large leaves are bright green on the top and whitish on the bottom due to fine hairs growing on the undersides. The leaves reach up to 12 inches long and are wider at the stem, tapering into a point. They are irregularly toothed on the edges and grow alternately up the stem. The single flower heads grow off small branches that come from the main stem. The flowers grow up to 2 inches wide and have a yellow disklike center that is velvety to the touch. From the disk, up to 100 bright yellow ray florets extend. There are multiple flowers on each plant.

Parts used: Roots, rhizomes, and flowers

Cautions: Occasional allergic reactions may occur. *Inula* should not be used during pregnancy or lactation. Diabetics should check blood sugars more often when using elecampane due to the inulin content.

Folklore and history: According to M. Grieve in *A Modern Herbal*, the name for this plant has many folktales attached to it, one of which is that the plant was created from the tears of Helen of Troy. Another folktale said that Helen of Troy used it against bites of poisonous serpents. Historically, the Greeks and Romans used elecampane as a cure-all for ailments ranging from dropsy, digestive upsets, and menstrual disorders to sciatica. By the nineteenth century, the herb was being used to treat skin disease, neuralgia, liver problems, and coughs. Elecampane's uses extended past medicinal, though, as it was used to add flavor to digestive liqueurs and vermouths. The herb was also candied and used in confectionery. People have used it as a cure for hydrophobia, or the fear of water, and for baby blessings.

Spiritual uses: Elecampane is an interesting plant because it is hard to pin down its magical uses. When I first started growing this plant, I went out and meditated with it, as I usually do, and I got some interesting results. To me, the plant feels very protective, standing like a sentry, straight and tall, with bright yellow flowers and leaves that resemble lungs. When I first connected with the plant on a spiritual level, I felt like it was a guardian plant, but not just a regular guardian; to me, it talked about being the guardian of the Breath of Life. Now, knowing what its medicinal uses were, I felt like I knew what it was talking about, but it seems that I only had part of the picture. It told me about being the guardian of the Breath of Life, which, to it, was not only the beginning of life but the beginning of universal power. It then told me that it could be used to either give individuals power or take that power away. This plant can be used in not only general protective magic, but it can also be used to protect your Breath of Life or personal power. This plant is a very sunny, happy plant; when people see its bounty of bright yellow flowers, it makes them smile and want to touch the plant. Now, given the lore that it sprung from Helen of Troy's tears, this indicates an ability to clear melancholy or sadness. I have also heard that the plant restores childlike joy to people who have forgotten their inner child.

Spiritual anecdote: I once had a client who had asthma and was depressed. Her asthma was made worse by stressful events in her life. When her boyfriend broke up with her and she was in crisis, I had her come to my house for an emergency balancing because her inhalers weren't working well. She came to the back door, where my treatment room was, and she saw the 6-foot-high elecampane plants I had growing. She first took a deep breath, then she smiled and said that she felt better just by looking at them. Now, I only use elecampane for lung infections, but her reaction to the plants gave me the knowledge that she needed them to help her heal. So, I added elecampane root tincture to her medicinal blend and called to check on her the next day. She said she felt much better and that she hadn't had to use her inhaler since she started taking the tincture. She also wasn't as upset about the breakup. She then made a comment that made me realize how important elecampane is for emotional distress; she told me that the tincture made her feel stronger and like she could get through her situation.

Astrological association: Mercury

Deities, angels, or spirit associations: Athena and Apollo

Meditation: Ray of sunshine, light my way into your warm and protective arms. Allow me to feel comfort, joy, and happiness in your presence.

Magical spell: To help someone who needs to have some joy brought back into their life, make an infused oil with the roots, add some essential oil (jasmine or ylang-ylang would be nice), and have the individual rub it on their hands as they say the plant's meditation.

Eyebright (*Euphrasia officinalis*)

Common names: Euphrasia, Euphrosyne, and red eyebright

Description: Eyebright is a small annual that can be found in meadows, pastures, and other grassy areas. Its square stem is covered in fine white hairs and grows to be 8 to 9 inches tall. Eyebright bears lanceolate, toothed leaves alternately along the stem, which are approximately ⅙ to ½ inch long and ⅓ inch wide. The small flowers come in white, red, or yellow. They are usually tinged with purple markings and have a yellow spot in the throat. The flowers are axillary and two lipped on the top and three lipped on the bottom with four stamens that protrude from the throat.

Parts used: Aerial parts

Cautions: None known; this plant is at risk for extinction due to over har-vesting, though. Please use it with the utmost respect.

Folklore and history: According to the doctrine of signatures and as stated by Gerard in *The Herbal*, "the purple and yellow spots and stripes of the Eyebright doth very much resemble the diseases of the eye, as bloodshot, by which signature it hath been found out that this herb is effectual in the curing of the same." In the highlands of Scotland, it was used as a cure for those who were almost blind by making an infusion in milk, soaking a feather in it, and dropping it into the eye. The Latin name for this herb, *Euphrasia*, is derived from the name of Zeus's daughter Euphrosyne, who was one of the three Graces. Euphrosyne was supposed to be the happi-est; she saw everything in the best light possible and gave the gift of joy and mirth to humankind, which is why the herb is named after her.

Spiritual uses: This herb is well known as an aid to help develop and strengthen psychic abilities, but if I had to describe this herb's magical affinities in two words, they would be *clear sight*. Now, what does this mean magically? Well, first the obvious: it helps with psychic abilities. It can be added to a divination tea, or one can make a cold infusion with which to wash the eyes prior to any major scrying or divination work. The phrase also means "the ability to see past obstacles or to see the larger picture that is often obscured." There are times when I need to see the hidden truths regarding a magical situation, and these are the times when I throw some eyebright on the coals and meditate on the big picture. So, eyebright can be used to see what is hidden either in the future, in the past, or in any situation. It also helps with seeing the opportunities in sometimes difficult situations. Sometimes all we can see are the things blocking us, but with eyebright, you can see beyond the obstacles, which can make the journey seem easier.

Spiritual anecdote: I use this sparingly in my divination tisane, mixing it with blue vervain, mugwort, and wild lettuce to make a drink that relaxes the mind, opens the third eye, and allows visions to come clearly. Once, I was selling teas and aromatherapy at a New Age fair, and my booth was surrounded by readers at tables. I had brewed a pot of divination tisane to give samples of at the event, and one of the mediums came up to me and asked about a drink her spirit guide had told her I made. She had been experiencing a dry spell for a while and had issues connecting with the Divine due to some personal stuff going on in her life. She was getting really worried because she wasn't making enough to pay the bills, which of course affected her ability to read even more. Her spirit guide had elbowed her and told her to come to me and ask for some of my special tisane, which I gave her to drink. What was interesting was that before I gave her the drink, she didn't have many customers, and after she drank the tisane, it got busy. She thanked me afterward and told me that she had made enough money that day to pay her rent, which took a lot of stress off her.

Astrological association: Mercury

Deities, angels, or spirit associations: Cerridwen, Herne, Hermes, and Euphrosyne

Meditation: Beautiful herb of sight, give me visions and make my path bright. Open the way so that I can see all that I need to be.

Magical spells: Make a tisane with equal parts mugwort, eyebright, and peppermint; add honey to taste, drink it, and then say the plant's meditation three times before using tarot cards or scrying with a crystal ball. It will help you get in the right space and clear your third eye to get the best vision. I also wash my crystal ball with the blend to help me see into it.

Fennel (*Foeniculum vulgare*)

Common names: Fenkel, finkle, and fennel fruit

Description: Fennel is a short-lived perennial or annual that can grow up to 3 feet tall and is grayish green in color. The stems grow alternately directly from the ground, forming an aboveground bulb with the shallow roots being underground. The stems are wider at the base (similar to celery) and grow narrower toward the top. The dark green, feathery leaves grow bilaterally from joints in the stem. The flowers are five-petaled and grow groups of four to thirty simple umbels, which are compounded into a larger umbel. The fruits are white to pale yellow, ovoid-oblong, and ridged. All parts of the plant contain the herb's characteristic licorice flavor.

Parts used: The fruit; the herb and fresh bulb can be cooked.

Cautions: None known

Folklore and history: Pliny, in his book *Natural History: A Selection*, recommended fennel for "dimness of vision," while Gerard wrote, "Fennel seede drunke assuageth the paine of the stomache, and the wambling of the same, or desire to vomite, and breaketh winde." It was believed to have magical powers in the Middle Ages and was hung over doors to keep out witches. It is also traditionally considered to be a remedy for snakebites. It is written that the Greeks used fennel stalks as staffs in parades dedicated to Dionysus and used the seeds to assist with flatulence after a large meal.

Spiritual uses: Purification, healing, protection, and removing obstacles; an herbal tea made from fennel, if drunk, will not only promote healing on the medicinal level, but it will also help promote spiritual healing, especially from psychic attacks. Burning fennel seeds in incense is wonderful for a simple purification ritual. When I need to remove obstacles in my life, I sprinkle some fennel seeds wherever the obstacle is. For example, if I am having money-related problems, I sprinkle some in my wallet and on my bank statement. I have also had them sitting at my desk in a bowl, and whenever I come across a problem that I don't know how to fix, I run my fingers through them and the answer to my issue comes to me. I love fennel because it's so small and inconspicuous that it can be added to potpourri or a small dish in an office or home and no one would know that you have a magical tool in your reach. The thing to remember with fennel seeds is that they have a strong licorice scent/taste; unless you love licorice, you may want to use them sparingly.

Spiritual anecdote: Once, I was trying to make the decision to leave my job at a hospital and transition to working in a clinic setting. I put a teaspoon of fennel seeds in a small organza bag and carried them in my pocket for about a week at work, occasionally handling them and inhaling their scent. A week later, I was looking at job advertisements at a local clinic, and I decided to apply. I ended up getting the job.

Astrological association: Mercury

Deities, angels, or spirit associations: Hermes, Michael the Archangel, Prometheus, Dionysus, and Artemis

Meditation: *Seed so small, seed so sweet, open my eyes to the clarity I seek.*

Magical spell: To attract money, buy a small green pouch and fill it with basil and fennel seeds. Say the plant's chant three times during the full moon and put the pouch in your purse or pocket.

Fig (*Ficus carica*)

Common names: Ficus, common fig, and flesh fruit

Description: The fig tree is an intriguing plant, botanically speaking. The leaves each have five lobes, which are about the size of a small hand and rough to the touch. The fig tree usually grows from 18 to 20 feet tall in warm climates, such as the western United States or the Mediterranean. The tree can be grown in colder climates if it is brought inside during the winter months. The fig itself is actually neither a fruit nor a flower but a little of both. The flowers reside inside a hollow, fleshy receptacle, which contains many small individual flowers. The edge of the receptacle curves inward, and it is on this part that the male flowers reside. The pollen from these flowers is then released inward to fertilize the inner flowers. This produces many one-seeded fruits that are contained within the original receptacle.

Parts used: Leaves and fruit

Cautions: None known

Folklore and history: In ancient Greece the fig was a symbol of fertility, prosperity, and strength; the best figs were saved for the gods, while nobility and the finest athletes received the next choice fruits. The fig also played into the worship of Bacchus and was used in religious rituals aimed at fertility of the people and their crops. This fruit was often dedicated to Bacchus because it was said that he introduced it to humankind. In rituals dedicated to him, the people of Cyrene would wear crowns of fig leaves as they went to the temples to leave him sacrifices.

Spiritual uses: The fig plant has great potential for magical use due to not only its leaf structure but because of the fruit's signature. The leaves, as I mentioned before, have five lobes, which look like a pentacle, so to me the leaves themselves are a perfect balance of all the elements plus Akasha, or spirit. This indicates that the leaves could be used in elemental workings or in any magical spell where perfect balance is required. The fruit and the way it reproduces is fascinating. To me, the fleshy cavity with the small flowers within it represents the womb. This, plus the way that the fruit is produced, is symbolic of not only fertility magic but of magic where one needs to journey within to accomplish a magical goal or dark moon magical workings. The milky sap of the fig tree can also be used in banishing magic. Grind figs up to use in incense for prosperity, fertility, and sensuality. I also use them in addition to dates in different types of Egyptian incense dedicated to Isis.

Spiritual anecdote: I remember doing a fertility ritual for a woman who was trying to conceive. She did every mundane thing possible—medications, insertion, in vitro—and nothing seemed to work. She and her husband had given up hope, and they were starting the adoption procedure. I balanced her hormones and uterus with herbal formulas, and then we did a ritual, which included her eating a fig. I also had her eat a fig every day to prepare for whatever was coming, whether it was a pregnancy or an adoption. Two months later I got a phone call from my client; she was so excited it was hard to understand her at first. She was pregnant—she had just had it confirmed by the doctor. I saw her the next week, and we worked on keeping her body strong with herbs through the pregnancy.

Astrological association: Jupiter

Deities, angels, or spirit associations: Bacchus, three Graces, Hera, Isis, and Persephone

Meditation: Fruit so round and plump, grant me the (riches, fertility, sensuality) I desire, and as I consume you, may you infuse your gifts into my being.

Magical spell: Take a fig and concentrate on what you are trying to achieve. Put that energy into the fig, and then eat it. As you eat it, the magic will be inside you.

Foxglove (*Digitalis purpurea*)

Common names: Dog's fingers, fairy caps, fairy fingers, fairy petticoats, fairy thimbles, fairy weed, floppy-dock, floptop, folk's-gloves, lady's-glove, plant of the fairy woman, virgin's glove, witches' bells, and witches' gloves

Description: Foxglove is a biennial that grows 3 feet tall on average and produces flowers in its second year on a red-streaked stem. In the first year, it grows narrow, bright green leaves in a rosette pattern. In its second year, the plant sends up a flower spike that reaches 1 to 2 feet long. The flowers bloom along the stem and vary in shade, ranging from a creamy white to a pale magenta color, with brown to black dots. The flowers are tubular and lipped with the lips sometimes being tinged a different color. The flowers hang downward, resembling a gloved finger, hence some of its common names.

Parts used: Leaves and flowers

Cautions: Do not take internally—this plant will cause poisoning, even in small doses. Do not burn in incense.

Folklore and history: There are many stories about how foxglove got its name, and if you look at the flowers, you can see why. According to European lore, foxglove was originally called "folk's-glove" because the flowers look like the fingers of a glove; it was said to be the glove of the fairy folk. One of the myths about how the name foxglove came about was that some fairies gave the flowers to a fox to protect his feet as he walked in brambles to do a favor for them. Another legend says the spots on the flowers were the fingerprints of elves after they had hidden themselves from human sight and that the spots were a path for bees to follow to get to the best nectar. There's also lore from Europe that says that if you play with foxglove flowers, you will become "fairy-struck". This lore was brought to the United States by Scottish families that settled in the Appalachians. Some of the older names reference the Virgin Mary, and these are often veiled references to older goddess worship. In Italian magical lore, the foxglove makes the intended open to sexual love.

Spiritual uses: If you haven't guessed it, foxglove is one of the favorite plants of the fey and a very magical plant. It is said that planting foxglove in your garden will attract all sorts of nature spirits, including elves and fairies. Foxglove can be used for protection, from both external and internal forces. I have foxglove planted along the walkway to my house as it makes a wonderful psychic/fairy barrier against people that would cause me harm. I plant it in my garden near my fairy houses so the fairies can hide in the flowers if someone were to walk by. I also cut a flower stalk of it to put on my altar when doing fairy magic.

Spiritual anecdote: I once had a client who kept having problems with missing objects. She once lost her car keys for two weeks and had to have a locksmith make new keys for her house and car. At first, she thought it was neighbor children sneaking in, and then she thought it was the stray cat she had been feeding that was taking her stuff. I had her take a stem of foxglove flowers from my garden and put it on the table in her kitchen. I told her to thank the fairies for visiting but that she needed her things back. Within two days her keys were found under the kitchen table and her other missing objects appeared nearby on a table.

Astrological association: Venus

Deities, angels, or spirit associations: Persephone, Hecate, the Virgin Mary, the fey/fairies, and the Queen of the Fairies

Meditation: Ancient plant of the fey, please help me find things in this time of need.

Magical spell: I grow it in my garden so that there is a safe place for the fey to hide if someone were to walk by, and I always dry a few of the flowers to put on my fairy altar as an offering.

Frankincense (*Boswellia sacra*)

Common names: Olibanum, horn of Africa, and Indian frankincense

Description: Frankincense is a tree native to Yemen, Saudi Arabia, Sudan, and Ethiopia that can grow up to 26 feet tall. It has a reddish middle bark with a papery, gray-colored outer bark. It's a deciduous tree that sheds its leaves in the winter. Its leaves are compound in nature with groupings of leaflets; the leaves themselves are leathery, medium green on the top, and grayish green on the bottom with a soft, velvety texture. The small flowers grow off new shoots that alternate along the branches. The flowers have five petals, which are white with a yellow tinge; the center of the flower is yellow with bright yellow anthers that fade to a light red. The seeds are teardrop shaped with several internal cupules. The sap is extracted by making small cuts in eight- to ten-year-old trees. The sap is allowed to harden on the trees over ten days, then the sap, which looks like tears, is collected over the summer season. As the summer lengthens, the purity of the frankincense tears increases until the sap becomes a cloudy blue color; this is considered the highest quality sap and is priced accordingly.

Parts used: Gum and essential oil

Cautions: None known

Folklore and history: This resin's use as incense has been documented as far back as the fifteenth century BC. The first records were found on an Egyptian temple dedicated to Queen Hatshepsut and discussed transporting resins, gold, and incense from a land called Punt, which historians believe was on the Horn of Africa or Ethiopia, via the Red Sea. Frankincense resin was probably used as a sacred offering, for mummification, and as medicine before these trades were documented.

It is heavily used in India during wedding ceremonies and as offerings during festivals of deities. In the Catholic church, it is used heavily at both Christmas and Easter, which are both celebratory times—one being the birth of Jesus and the other the rebirth of Jesus.

Spiritual uses: Purification, protection, and removing negative spirits or demons; it can also be used as an offering, especially to Egyptian, Sumerian, or many Middle Eastern deities, or as a blessing herb. I consider frankincense to be one of my most important resins to use for purification, and I often use it to purify a space before a ritual, for house purifications, and for house blessings.

Spiritual anecdote: I once went to a house that was reputed to be haunted and performed a house blessing, using frankincense in large amounts. The house's owner was a medium and was okay with the spirits there because they were twins who had died as children from respiratory infections and were not harmful. So, instead of using an herbal wand or palo santo, which would drive a spirit out, I used straight frankincense. The medium said she felt the children try to hide from the incense but only because they didn't like the smell; since they were innocent children, they were not affected by its ability to remove negative spirits. After that day the medium said that every time the children started getting mischievous (hiding items), she burned frankincense, and they went to what was their playroom to hide and behaved for a period of time.

Astrological association: Sun

Deities, angels, or spirit associations: Inanna, Sekhmet, Anubis, and Ra

Meditation: Ancient tree, lend the power of your lifeblood to purify me.

Magical spell: Frankincense resin can always be burned in incense, but I like to put a bag with a piece of frankincense and a few crystals in my car's glove box for protection. For me it's used as protection against getting a speeding ticket and to keep the spirits I clean from houses from following me home. If you're prone to getting speeding tickets, you can carry frankincense and crystals in your vehicle to do the same.

Galangal (*Alpinia galanga*)

Common names: Greater galangal, *lengkuas*, blue ginger, *laos*, chewing John, High John the Conqueror, and court case root

Description: Galangal is a member of the ginger family, and they have similar characteristics. The parts used are the rhizomes and roots, which spread by underground runners. The roots are thick, white, and covered with a very brown skin. The stems, which can reach 6 feet tall, grow from eyes in the rhizomes, and as they age, the number of eyes increases. The leaves grow off the stems in an alternating pattern. The leaves are large, sometimes 2 feet long, lance shaped, and medium green with deep veins the same color as the leaves. The flowers come from the tops of the leaf stems, are white with thin pink stripes, and have three petals and two stamens that self-pollinate the flower. The red fruit produced is small and has a single seed in it.

Parts used: Roots and rhizomes

Cautions: None known

Folklore and history: Historically, galangal has mostly been used as a spice in Indian, Southeast Asian, and some African cuisine. It is a medicinal herb in Unani medicine. Hildegard von Bingen, an abbess and author, called it a medicine of the heart in *Hildegard von Bingen's Physica* and wrote that "whoever has pain in the heart area or is suffering weakness due to the heart, should immediately eat enough galangal and he will recover." There is also history in voodoo about the root; in voodoo galangal is also called High John the Conqueror, who is said to be a spirit who came to North America with the enslaved people to protect them. Once slavery ended, he went into the roots of the plant to help people with their problems.

Spiritual uses: Galangal is known for its ability to win court cases, but it is also a protective herb against hexes and curses. It can also be used to strengthen the heart, which to me means it gives courage to the user and helps them get through hard times. One of galangal's lesser-known abilities is being able to increase a magical formula's power if a little of the plant is added to the mix.

Spiritual anecdote: I had an herbal client once who got tangled up with a bad business partner who left her with lots of legal troubles, including more than twenty lawsuits against her and the business. She told me that she won all of the court issues against her not only because she kept good records, but because she always carried galangal root with her into court. She was still afraid, though. Her fear was that because her business partner had swindled so many people, she would always be called into court, and all of the stress from these legal battles was wearing on her health. I worked with her to use her magical practices and galangal root to heal her spiritual field, as well as her physical body, and increase her courage. I did this by instructing her to grow a patch of galangal in her garden. As she tended it and the patch grew, she grew healthier. An interesting side effect was that she did not have as many lawsuits.

Astrological associations: Moon and Mars

Deities, angels, or spirit associations: The apostles and Justicia

Meditation: *Sacred root of High John the Conqueror, please help me obtain justice in my court case; protect me against unjust actions.*

Magical spell: Take a slice of the root, put it in a red bag, say the plant's meditation, and carry the bag with you to the courthouse to help you have favorable outcomes in court.

Garlic (*Allium sativum*)

Common names: Stinking radish, poor man's treacle, camphor of the poor, nectar of the gods, and stinking rose

Description: The leaves are long, green, and somewhat flat, and the small, whitish flowers grow from a central stem and are arranged in an umbel shape. The bulb is compound, subspherical, and covered with membranous whitish scales. About ten wedge-like, compressed cloves are arranged circularly around a central stem base. The smaller cloves surround those laterally and are each separated by the whitish scale. Each clove is covered by its own thinner scale, which is often removed before cooking.

Parts used: Bulbs

Cautions: Large doses cause nausea, vomiting, and purging; it can also change the odor of milk if breastfeeding. It can lower blood sugar, so those with hypoglycemia should check their blood sugars more frequently unless large amounts of garlic are part of their normal diet. Garlic can also cause insomnia or aldosterone insufficiency in large amounts. Those with impending surgery or taking blood thinners should also use it in moderation internally.

Folklore and history: Garlic was a valuable medicine in ancient Greece, Rome, China, and Egypt, and in *Natural History*, Pliny the Elder recommended garlic for more than sixty uses, including treating wounds from animals and as an antidote to henbane poisoning. Sailors, Roman soldiers, and medieval knights used it as a protective amulet in battle. It was also used as an aphrodisiac, and an old Italian piece of lore says that a woman who cooks with lots of garlic will never have her husband looking for another lover. In some European and Hungarian lore, it was said that competitors would not be able to outrun someone who chewed a clove while running a race, and it is still used in some Hungarian horse races as people keep a garlic clove tucked somewhere on the horse to give it an edge over its competitors.

There is a long history of garlic being offered to Hecate, either during rites or as an offering left at crossroads. In the temples of Cybele, a person who had eaten garlic was not allowed entrance.

Spiritual uses: Protection is one of garlic's main uses, and a bulb placed at all four corners of a house is said to keep away diseases, including the plague. It is also said that one can chase away evil spirits and multiple monsters simply by placing garlic around the house or by biting into it. I plant it along my garden borders not only to discourage deer and rabbits but to keep negative energy or people from my land. If you know someone is causing you harm, I advise you to write their name on a clove of garlic and to put the clove in a window or by the front door. It will stop that individual in their tracks, and they will not be able to harm you.

Spiritual anecdote: I have used garlic against psychic vampires—you know the kind. Sometimes you feel spaced-out or weak around them, but when they finally leave, you feel drained of your energy or sick. I once had a friend who was a psychic vampire but didn't know it. I would spend time with her, and soon after we would part ways, I would feel exhausted and sick. I started carrying a clove of garlic when I visited her to test my theory. Lo and behold, I felt better, and she had to cut our visit short because she started having some indigestion. Soon afterward I talked to her and trained her (over the phone at first) how to stop draining energy from others. Once she was aware of what she was doing, she was able to mostly stop.

I also have recommended garlic to people who have vampiric coworkers they can't escape from. I tell them to put a clove in their desk for a week at a time (replacing it weekly so that it remains strong). It keeps the energy sucker away—and all kinds of other negativity as well.

Astrological association: Mars

Deities, angels, or spirit associations: Hecate, Athena, and Zeus

Meditation: *Bulb so strong, protect me from all those who wish me harm.*

Magical spell: It's easy to slip a garlic clove into a small bag or hide a clove in your home somewhere for protection, but I tell people to change it every week because the clove will absorb negativity and rot in half the time it is supposed to. Also, the scent is what repels negativity and harm, so a fresh clove will work better.

Ginseng (*Panax* spp.)

Common names: Five-finger plant, manroot, redberry, sang, tartar root, and wonder of the world root

Description: Ginseng grows in humus-rich forests with thick leaf canopies. The plant grows on a series of 1- to 2-foot-long stalks that send out branches at almost 45-degree angles and produce leaves that are 5 to 7

inches long. These leaves are oblong in shape and medium green in color with a double-toothed edge. They grow in threes, each divided into five sections. The flowers are small, white, and grow in umbel groupings. The bright red berries produced are also small, and within each fruit are two seeds. The root is the part that is used medicinally, and it is yellowish white and slightly fleshy in texture. Ginseng roots are unique in that they often resemble the human body or a body part.

Parts used: Roots

Cautions: Ginseng should not be taken if you are pregnant, if you have high blood pressure, or with other stimulants, such as caffeine. Ginseng is at risk of extinction due to overharvesting; substitute with Solomon's seal or May apple.

Folklore and history: Ginseng was one of the first herbs documented, and it was written about in ancient Chinese and Greek materia medicas as a miracle herb that could rebalance, recharge, and make the weak strong again. It was used in eastern Asia for everything from skin conditions to impotence.

There are several types of plants that make up the ginseng family; *Panax quinquefolium*, or American ginseng, and *Panax ginseng*, or Asian ginseng, are the two most common. Some plants were historically called ginseng, such as Siberian ginseng, but were not true *Panax* species. They were later renamed to define this difference.

Spiritual uses: Ginseng can be used in several types of workings, mostly because of its human shape and ability to enhance sexual performance. I have used ginseng roots to represent body parts in healing spells, and it works quite well. I usually infuse the root with the energy that is needed. I then give it to the person that needs it and have them wear it, carry it, or ingest it. Ginseng is also one of the only substitutes for whole mandrake root due to its ability to look like the human body.

In South Korea, where I was stationed for a year during my time with the United States military, I met a root doctor who cured people with ginseng roots. They would come in and tell him what was wrong, and he would either sell them a dried root out or liquor with a fresh root steeped in it. The roots he used would often resemble the organ that was causing the issue.

When I lived in upstate New York, I was good friends with a Santería priestess. One night she was going to do some hex-breaking magic against someone who was trying to harm her magically, so she went into the forest and came out with this root that looked like a person. The root was American ginseng. Her comment was that sure, she could make a poppet, but if you *really* wanted the job done right, there nothing was better than a poppet made by nature herself.

Spiritual anecdote: I have used ginseng several times, mostly for healing, but because of its endangered status and high cost, I do not use it often. I was fortunate enough to live in Minnesota, which is close enough in proximity to some large American ginseng farms, and I was able to get a pound of fresh root for a reasonable price. In this batch of white American ginseng, there was a root that looked like lovers entwined. I made a tincture from it and used it in my herbal practice to help with sexual problems, ranging from impotence to infertility. I also sprinkled this tincture on poppets and spell bags to assist with sexual disorders or relationship problems.

Astrological association: Sun

Deities, angels, or spirit associations: Quan Yin and the Guardians of the Four Quarters

Meditation: Man root, help me in my quest for sexual love and help stoke the fires of never-ending happiness.

Magical spell: For passionate love, take a red poppet or small bag and sprinkle the tincture of ginseng on it while saying the plant's chant. Carry the poppet or bag with you to attract sexual love.

Goldenseal (*Hydrastis canadensis*)

Common names: Eyebalm, eyeroot, ground raspberry, ghost plant, jaundice root, orangeroot, and yellowroot

Description: Goldenseal is an inconspicuous little plant that grows in moist, shaded forests and often in colonies. The root is the part that is most used medicinally, but there are some cases where the leaves have been used. The root is yellow and grows horizontally with thin rootlets that grow off the bottom and sides of the main root branch. The plant bursts from the ground in late April or early May. The leaves then unfurl from the top of the stem; they are dark green in appearance with deeply cut veins. The leaves have five lobes with the center three being the most pronounced and the lower two being less distinct. The leaves can grow from 4 to 10 inches wide. The flower is small, white or pink in color, and falls away soon after it opens, leaving multiple stamens. The berry that emerges is raspberry shaped. Each drupe contains one or two seeds that are hard and black.

Parts used: Roots and leaves

Cautions: Use in moderation; too much goldenseal root can cause high blood pressure. This plant is also endangered. If you must use it, use the leaf. Do not wildcraft goldenseal; buy it from an ethical source instead.

Folklore and history: There is a fair amount of Native American folklore about this plant. Some Indigenous peoples would use the leaves or roots as a wash or paint before hunting or battle to give themselves courage and to help keep themselves safe, and some tribes believed that a wash of the leaves alone would make a person undetectable to animals. One of the names my Dakota shaman teacher, Dottie Running Horse, called goldenseal was "ghost plant" because a shaman could make themselves invisible to both people and animals by snuffing the root.

Spiritual uses: Goldenseal leaves or roots can be added to a bath for purification and healing. Snuffing a pinch of goldenseal is supposed to make you invisible to animals and to people who are seeking to harm you. It is also used to attract money. Just put some leaves in your wallet to bring money to you.

Spiritual anecdote: Because it is endangered, I use goldenseal root mostly for healing work, but I once added the leaf to an invisibility blend I made for a teenager who was getting picked on at school. I added goldenseal leaf, agrimony, and mistletoe to a small bag and had the teen carry it to school. That stopped the bullying, and the teenager said that when he walked by the bullies, it was like they didn't even see him.

Astrological association: Sun

Deities, angels, or spirit associations: Michael the Archangel, Apollo, and Loki

Meditation: Root so golden, bring to me your ability to be financially free (or invisible) so that I may do what I need to do to be happy.

Magical spell: Mix a combination of equal parts agrimony, goldenseal leaf, and mistletoe together. Put the combination in a light purple bag, and carry it with you to help create a glamor of invisibility.

Hawthorn (*Crataegus oxyacantha*)

Common names: May blossom, quickthorn, whitethorn, haw, hagthorn, and ladies' meat, bread, and cheese tree

Description: Hawthorn, which is part of the rose family, is a hedgerow bush that can be trained into a small tree and grow up to 20 feet tall. The rough bark is grayish brown. There is a single trunk that comes out of the ground, and the branches start forming close to the base of the tree. The branches are uniform, heavily thorned, and evenly distributed up the trunk. The leaves are medium green in color with green veins. Each leaf has one or more lobes, and the edges grow in a dentate fashion. The flowers are small and white with five petals that come together at the base at the corolla, which is initially yellow. There are two short stamens per petal. Once the flower is pollinated, the corolla turns red. The berry, also called a haw, is small and red with a star-shaped crown on one end. It is attached to the branch with a red stem. The red berry has only one seed that can be medium or large in size relative to the size of the fruit.

Parts used: Leaves, flowers, and berries

Cautions: Can lower blood pressure when taken internally

Folklore and history: One of the legends about hawthorn is that the thorny branches formed the crown of thorns worn by Jesus at his crucifixion. Another legend, which originated in Glastonbury, England, says that Joseph of Arimathea planted his staff in the ground on the tor and the first hawthorn tree in the United Kingdom grew from his staff. That original tree had cuttings taken from it before a religious zealot burned it down. The trees grown from those cuttings were owned by the Queen of

England, and the blossoms were brought to her every year as part of the May Day festivals.

The deity most associated with the hawthorn tree is Cardea. As the myth behind it goes, Janus was enamored with her beauty, and in exchange for her virginity, he made her the goddess of hinges and gave her the hawthorn tree, which was used to repel evil spirits from passing through doorways. According to Ovid, a Roman poet, Cardea used the thorns of the tree to protect young children from evil spirits, called tristes, who sucked the blood from infants.

There are quite a few Beltane folk stories related to the flowers. It is said that at the dawning of Beltane, the women would gather the dew off the blossoms and wash their faces with it to stay looking young. A common custom was for a young man to give a bunch of hawthorn flowers to the one he desired on Beltane. If she accepted the flowers, they were a couple until the next Beltane.

Spiritual uses: Protection of infants and doorways, fertility, love, lust, and sexual rituals; it also restores or maintains youth.

Spiritual anecdote: I had a friend who had this beautiful piece of land in Wisconsin. She was planning on building a spiritual retreat on it, but since the land had been unused for more than a decade, the local hunters and teenage kids had taken to hunting and four-wheeling on it. She had tried talking to the locals, but they considered it theirs since the prior owner had died and my friend did not claim it right way. I walked the land with her, and in the middle of an open field was a giant hawthorn bush. My friend thought that this plant was the heart of the land; she wanted to make an offering to it but did not know how to do it. I had her bring some crystals, some incense, some flowers, and some fruit as an offering in the fall. The tree was covered with berries but also had mold and severe insect damage on the leaves. It felt like the tree was dying because the land was neglected. We left the offerings to the tree so that it would heal and also so it would protect the land from the people who were damaging the earth with their four-wheelers. The following May we came back to see that the tree was filled with blossoms, the bark was free from mold, and the land where the four-wheelers had been causing damage was filled with hundreds of flowers and baby hawthorn trees.

Astrological association: Mars

Deities, angels, or spirit associations: Cardea, Persephone, and Janus

Meditation: On Beltane, say: *Flower, musky and sweet, help me attract my one true love to me today and until the love fades.*

Magical spell: For protection, take equal parts dried hawthorn berries, frankincense, and cedar wood and grind them together, concentrating on your intention to protect your home/family. Begin burning a charcoal and put the dried herb combination on it. Burn the incense as you walk from outside your home to the inside while concentrating on protecting your home and allowing no one inside who wishes to harm you.

Henbane (*Hyoscyamus niger*)

Common names: Hyoscyami folium, black henbane, Devil's eyes, fetid night shade, henbell, hog's-bean, Jupiter's-bean, poison tobacco, stinking nightshade, symphonica, cassilato, and cassilago

Description: Henbane is a slightly sticky, hairy biennial. A rosette of basal leaves grows in the first year, followed in the second year by an erect, simple or slightly branched stem that grows 1 to 2 feet tall and is covered with sticky hairs. The alternate leaves are oval, deeply toothed, and pinnately lobed to indented. Sessile flowers grow from the axils of the leaves and have bell-shaped petals, which run into five pointed tips, and tube-like, yellow, externally hairy, fused-at-the-base corollas, which have violet veins that start that the tip of the petals and travel deep into the violet mouth. The fruit capsules contain up to five hundred grayish-brown seeds. All parts of the plant are poisonous. The taste and odor are unpleasant.

Parts used: Leaves

Cautions: It is very poisonous; do not eat, burn as incense, or drink.

Folklore and history: Henbane has long been associated with Witchcraft, magical spells, and fortune-telling. Henbane's aphrodisiac properties were written about in Gerard's *Herbal*, and he discussed its use in love potions. The Oracle of Delphi was thought to inhale the burning root of henbane in addition to the volcanic fumes to prophesize for kings and travelers who came for answers. The Greeks believed that people who inhaled or ate henbane became prophetic and that the madness that happened was part of the gift the gods gave the people. In Greek mythology, the dead in Hades were crowned with a wreath of henbane as they wandered along the Styx. In Shakespeare's *Hamlet*, Hamlet's father comes back as a ghost and says that he was murdered when the juice of henbane was poured in his ear by Claudius.

Spiritual uses: I use henbane in external magical ointments to help with divination, trance work, and pain relief. I put it in gris-gris bags, along with other love-attracting herbs, for love and aphrodisiac spell work.

Spiritual anecdote: I once had a friend who was a bit of an artist; the problem was that she was afraid she wasn't good enough, and her fear kept her from becoming as great as she could be. Her lack of confidence and self-love was her greatest obstacle, and she knew it. So, we made a charm to help her love herself, increase her confidence in her work, and put her on the right path that included henbane, a gold-colored coin, and a piece of rose quartz. Within six months she had her first gallery opening, and now she is a well-known painter in New York City, where she lives.

Astrological association: Saturn

Deities, angels, or spirit associations: Hades, Hecate, Ganesh, Isis, and Belenus

Meditation: Mistress of wisdom, guide me to my desires; show me the way to my desires.

Magical spell: Take a piece of the root, and while saying the plant's meditation, place it in a charm bag. Carry the bag with you to open new paths and to help guide you to your destiny.

Holly (*Ilex aquifolium*)

Common names: Aquifolius, bat's wings, Christ's-thorn, holy tree, holme chaste, hulm, and hulver bush

Description: A large shrub or small tree with smooth, light gray bark, holly has leaves that are dark green and glossy. The leaves are approximately 2 inches long and stiff when you try to bend them. The leaves have alternating thorny spines on the borders. Holly has small white flowers, which bloom in the spring, and produces small bright red berries in the fall. The berries are toxic to ingest, and it's the leaves that are actually used in modern herbalism. The berries and bark can be used magically or as altar decorations as long as they are not eaten.

Parts used: Leaves, berries, and bark

Cautions: Some species of holly leaves contain caffeine; if ingesting the leaves as a tisane, know if you are drinking a caffeinated or non-caffeinated member of the family. The berries are toxic; do not ingest them.

Folklore and history: Since the time of the Druids, holly has been seen as an herb of protection. The Druids used the evergreen branches as protection in their homes and sacred spaces, and they also used holly to create a safe space for nature spirits to live during the winter. It's believed that a holly plant grown near a house will protect it from lightning, poison, and negative magic. According to Pliny the Elder, planting holly next to a house protected the home and its inhabitants from lightning, poisoning, and Witchcraft. It was also used to keep animals from fleeing. If an animal did start to run away, a holly stick was thrown after it, and this caused the creature to return to the owner. Holly is well known in magical circles as a Yule-time plant that represents the god as he makes his ascent from the underworld to be reborn from the goddess.

Spiritual uses: Protection, luck, attracting money, and good fortune spell work; I always hang holly branches above my door (along with evergreens and ivy) to welcome in good fortune and the blessings of the god and goddess for the New Year. I also give holly plants to friends that are in need of a little extra good fortune or protection during the Yule season.

Spiritual anecdote: I had a friend who was going through a horrible time. She had lost her job, and her husband had left her. She felt scared because she was all alone with no money. A few of us got together as a support group. I brought some holly branches, another friend brought grapevine, and another friend brought pine and fir boughs. Together we cast a circle and did a magical working in which we, as a circle of friends, wove the holly, grapevine, and evergreens into a wreath for her to place over her door. This wreath was to offer her protection and to encourage good luck and fortune to come through her door. Less than a week later, she got a job offer from a great firm, and she got an unexpected check from a bank account she had closed years earlier.

Astrological association: Mars

Deities, angels, or spirit associations: Diana, the fey, and centaurs

Meditation: Herb so bright and evergreen, bring me all of the things to protect me.

Magical spell: Collect a good amount of holly branches and weave a portion of them into a round wreath to bring in wealth and good fortune. Weave the remaining branches into a pentacle for protection. Chant the plant's meditation three times, then hang the branches above the front door. It is best to hang one pentacle over each doorway to keep harmful influences from entering.

Hops (*Humulus lupulus*)

Common name: Beer flower

Description: Hops is a vining perennial that can grow as tall as 15 feet in perfect conditions. The leaves are dark green in color, heart shaped, and triple lobed, and they have deep veins with a sandpaper-like texture. The stems are nondescript, except for their stickiness, which allows them to attach to just about anything. The flowers are inside a cone-shaped catkin called a strobile, which is the most distinguishing part of the plant. They are a pale yellow green and cone shaped with many petals that loosely shelter the center flower/fruit. The female flowers contain a yellow substance called lupulin, which is one of its active ingredients. Each plant produces male or female flowers, both of which are used in brewing and lose effectiveness with storage.

Parts used: Flowers or strobiles

Cautions: Do not drink an herbal tea made from hops when on antidepressants or pain killers; it may intensify their effects.

Folklore and history: Hops is a wonderful plant that, as many know, is used to give bitterness to beer. According to M. Grieve in *A Modern Herbal*, the use of hops in brewing ale was only documented as early as the fourteenth century. Prior to that, other herbs, such as ground ivy, were used as bitters. Hops were used as bitters because the plant was known to be an anti-aphrodisiac and was added to the beers of monks so that they would not wish to procreate. The Romans ate the young shoots of the hops plant as a bitter to help with digestion.

Spiritual uses: I have found that hops can be used for several magical purposes. The plant is extremely stubborn and can grow in a variety of conditions and still thrive. The plant also has the ability to climb just about anything. To me, this points to its ability to help you overcome obstacles that you might not even realize are there. Because hops is a nervine, it has sedative properties that can assist with divination when mixed with other herbs, such as mugwort, yarrow, or lavender. You could either put some of this herb in a dream pillow or have a cup of tea made with it before bed to help you see the future in your dreams. I often stuff hops into pillows to promote peaceful sleep and prophetic dreams. I also use it to help people see the obstacles that they can't see when they are awake and fully conscious; it allows the unconscious to unlock itself from the day-to-day and shows the way toward a clear path.

Spiritual anecdote: I had a friend who needed guidance with a marriage issue. It was hard for her to make the decision to leave him because there were children involved. Using hops, I made her a pillow for her to sleep on as well as a tincture to help her find her true path in life. The tools helped her see that while the relationship was to end, the other person had come to the same conclusion she had. After two weeks she had a conversation with her partner, and they worked out a friendly separation. They parted as friends, and in the end they became better people and parents.

Astrological associations: Mars and Pluto

Deities, angels, or spirit associations: Pan and Saint Martin of Tours, who rules monks

Meditation: *Herb so dreamy, help me open my mind and my heart to my true destiny and help me remove the blocks in my way.*

Magical spell: Sew some hops into a small pillow. Place this pillow in your pillowcase with the intent of giving you visions that will help you see any obstacles in your life. If you do not know how to sew, a sock or nylon knee-high can be stuffed with the herb and knotted at the end to keep the herb contained.

Horsetail (*Equisetum arvense*)

Common names: Bottle brush, Dutch rushes, paddock pipes, pewter-wort, and shave grass

Description: When horsetail first comes out of the ground, it appears like a single, medium green shoot that has nodular joints. The stem is hollow except for a thin membrane that sits in the joints of the plant. This membrane holds nutrient-rich fluid. Once the plant matures, it sends out fernlike leaves that come right off the joints and at the end, giving it the appearance of a horse's tail. Horsetail grows in swamp-like conditions, and it is often found on the edges of marshes and streams, usually growing in sandy soil. It is best harvested in the late spring, before it gets its leaves.

Parts used: Stems

Cautions: Ingesting too much horsetail can cause an electrolyte imbalance.

Folklore and history: Horsetail is an incredible plant that has been in existence since the time of the dinosaurs. During that time period, it is estimated that horsetail grew to be the size of a California redwood. In medieval Europe some of the larger species have been said to be used as broomsticks for witches. According to M. Grieve, soldiers used horsetail for centuries to stanch bleeding wounds and to help them heal as recently as the US Civil War. In India the plant was used to create a whistle to charm snakes.

Spiritual uses: Magically, this plant has a lot of possibilities that we can see just by observing it. First of all, horsetail can be used to increase fertility because if it is planted in a damp area, it will quickly take over and become invasive. Horsetail is also a tough plant, which means that it can be used to strengthen any spell. It also helps in breaking open both internal and external obstacles, especially when it comes to spiritual growth. Horsetail pipes have been used in the past to charm snakes, and this tells me that it can be used to charm both human and beast. In addition, this herb can be used in love and lust spells, especially when there are obstacles in the way.

Spiritual anecdote: I had a client who had a variety of issues, including an inability to fall in love. This had been a problem for her since both her father and her uncle had abused her. She was unable to love anything— food, puppies, and so on—and she had found this wonderful man whom she wanted to love but couldn't. So, we made some herbal combinations for her medical issues, and I added horsetail to the blend because she had this internal obstacle that she wanted removed. It took a few months of drinking horsetail tisane while she worked on balancing her chakras and meditating, but eventually she was able to love a dog. About a year later, she started falling in love with her long-term boyfriend.

Astrological association: Saturn

Deities, angels, or spirit associations: Epona, Pan, Macha, and Minoan Snake Goddess

Meditation: Allow your hollow stems to act as a pathway for me to obtain (insert whatever you need).

Magical spell: To help someone get through any obstacles they are experiencing, put horsetail in a small bag or in a tea, saying the plant's meditation.

Iris (*Iris versicolor*)

Common names: Blue flag, poison flag, flag lily, liver lily, and snake lily

Description: Iris versicolor grows from spreading rhizomes, which are dark brown on the outside and reddish white on the inside. The plants grow to be at least 31 inches tall. The stems grow from the eyes on the rhizomes, and the leaves grow in basal patterns along the stems. The leaves look like thick blades of grass, but they are actually folded over the middle vein or rib. The leaves are wider at the base and grow to a point, giving them a fanlike look. They are medium green in color. The flowers grow on stems that come from the rhizomes, and they have six crinkly petals and sepals that lie almost flat. Their color varies from a light blue to a deep blue, but it is not uncommon to get purple flowers. The throat of the flower is a greenish yellow to yellow. The fruit is in an angular capsule, and the seeds are large, medium brown, and can float on the air.

Parts used: Flowers and rhizomes

Cautions: Iris roots may be poisonous if ingested.

Folklore and history: The flower was named after the goddess of the rainbow, Iris, who brought the messages of the gods to humans. In some lore she is said to glide down a rainbow that she created to bring those messages. She also carried water from the river Styx to the gods for them to use. The iris is dedicated to Juno and is said to be the origin of the royal scepter. The iris was also used as a symbol to denote royalty and is seen throughout Europe on castles.

Spiritual uses: Communication, receiving messages from the gods, and fulfilling wishes

Spiritual anecdote: I had a client who grew the most beautiful iris plants. She had recently lost her husband, and she was quite distraught because he was an atheist and she, a Catholic, was afraid that he would be in purgatory for the rest of eternity. I went to her house and instructed her to pick three iris flowers, which I then had her place on a table in her living room. I proceeded to do a reading for her to see if we could figure out where he was. As I was laying out the cards, a wind came through the house and blew the vase over. Two of the flowers landed on the floor, but one of the flowers flew a little farther, coming to rest on her late husband's chair. At that point she started crying and told me that she had been thinking about throwing out his favorite chair. I realized that the reason the flower floated to the chair was that he was sending her a message that he was okay. I told her this and said that he was probably still hanging around because he was concerned about her. I then had her light a candle, held her hand, and had her talk to him to let him know that she was doing all right and that she missed him. After that I helped him with the transition to the other side. My client felt a lot of relief following that ritual, and she was able to get rid of his chair a few months later.

Astrological association: Venus

Deities, angels, or spirit associations: Hera and Iris

Meditation: *Iris, please help me communicate my desires to the gods so that they can make my wish come true.*

Magical spell: To make a wish come true, say the plant's meditation while burning incense with iris in it. Make sure to make an offering of bread, honey, or a coin to the deity Iris so that she will be more likely to grant your wish.

Ivy, Common (*Hedera helix*)

Common names: Ivy and Hedera

Description: Ivy is an evergreen, vining plant that can grow up to 98 feet long, especially if it has rocky cliffs or trees to attach to. Small rootlets grow along the vine in order to cling to any available surfaces. The palmate leaves grow alternating along the stem and have three main lobes, each of which end at a rounded point. The leaves are glossy, dark green with a light green center vein, and can grow to be 4 inches wide. Ivy has small, whitish-green, five-petaled flowers that grow at the end of the stem in an umbel pattern. Ivy produces a purple-black berry in the autumn that has several small black seeds in it.

Parts used: Leaves

Cautions: None known

Folklore and history: The ivy plant has been used in ritual and worship since the time of the Greeks and is associated with several deities. According to M. Grieve's *A Modern Herbal*, the Greeks wove it into crowns given to newlyweds to represent fidelity and into the crowns of the victorious at the Olympic Games. Ivy was also woven into the crowns of poets as they sang of the great feats of the gods and heroes. Ivy was heavily associated with Bacchus and Dionysus, and you can see it in the art from that period and the Renaissance where these images were popular. It was thought that ivy leaves could cure drunkenness, so Greeks used to boil ivy leaves in large vats of wine and decorate their ritual items with it.

Spiritual uses: Worship of Greek deities, fidelity, love, lust, and reducing addictions

Spiritual anecdote: I have used ivy in several sabbat rituals and handfastings as symbols of love, but once I had someone who wanted to stop drinking but was having a hard time doing it. He had joined AA, had a sponsor, was attending meetings, and had tried to stop his drinking multiple times with no luck. Because of this he asked me to perform a ritual to help him. For this ritual, I bound his hands with ivy vines and asked the plant to keep him from desiring alcohol and asked his personal deity to protect him against situations that may lead him to drinking again. After the ritual, I made an herbal tea of lemon balm, ivy, and peppermint for him to drink whenever he felt the urge to consume alcohol, and as of this writing, he has been sober for more than twenty years.

Astrological association: Saturn

Deities, angels, or spirit associations: Dionysus, Attis, and Cybele

Meditation: To help recover from an alcohol addiction, say: *Ivy vine, bind my desires and make me immune from the desires of alcohol.*

Magical spell: Mix ivy leaves, grape leaves, and mastic together and burn on coals as an offering of incense to the Greek gods. Carry the blend to add mirth and laughter to your life.

Ivy, Ground (*Glechoma hederacea*)

Common names: Creeping Charlie, over-the-gill, alehoof, gill-over-the-ground, tun-hoof, haymaids, hedgemaids, lizzy-run-up-the-hedge, robin-run-in-the-hedge, cat's-foot, cat's-paw, and gillrun

Description: Ground ivy is a creeping, rooting perennial that's common in most parts of the world. It's often found in woods, shady meadows, and damp fields, growing close to the ground and spreading by sending out runners that sink shallow roots into the ground. It is an invasive species in some regions and can take over a small space quickly if not monitored. The square stems are hairy, unbranched, and often reddish purple. The dark green, kidney-shaped leaves, which are opposite of one another, are up to 1 inch long, hairy, and serrated. The shoots off the stem bear pairs of two-lipped, pale violet flowers with dark purple spots from March to June in the axils of leaflike bracts. When crushed it has the smell of balsam.

Parts used: Aerial parts

Cautions: None known

Folklore and history: According to M. Grieve, ground ivy was first brought to the United States in the 1700s as a ground cover for semi-shady areas where grass wouldn't grow; today it is listed as a noxious weed. The Latin name is based on both the Greek word *glechon*, which means "ivy," and the Roman word *hedra*, which means "mint," so its name means "ivy like mint." The ancient Greeks were aware of its many powers and used it to ensure fertility, fidelity, and prosperity. According to Gerard, ground ivy was one of the plants used by the Saxons to purify and clarify their beer, and one of this plant's older names is alehoof for that reason. Ground ivy also acted as a preservative for the beer on long sea voyages. It was such a good preservative because the plant contains vitamin C and other nutrients.

Spiritual uses: Ground ivy is a weed of fertility, because as every gardener knows, it is impossible to get rid of. A little piece left in the ground will produce many offsprings in a short period of time. Ground ivy can also be carried to create either money or luck; it seems to draw money out of thin air when used in prosperity magic. Ground ivy can also be used as a protective herb. I have it growing everywhere in my front yard, and I have asked the spirit of the plant to be one of my protective allies. I have full confidence that if someone who wished me harm were to come up my walkway, this herb would protect me. It is an herb of alchemical properties, and it can change situations quickly.

Spiritual anecdote: This plant is one of my magical allies. I once had an individual visit my house who was not such a good person. He was coming over to tell me how he was right about something, how another was lying to me and should be banished from the Craft. As he walked up my sidewalk, he tripped twice. When he got to my door, he told me that some weeds on my path had tripped him. Needless to say, I understood what the ground ivy was trying to do. The plants were giving me a warning that this was a bad person, and they actually tried to stop him twice as he walked to my front door. I did not welcome him in when I realized he was out to cause me harm.

Astrological association: Venus

Deities, angels, or spirit associations: Diana, Epona, and Pan

Meditation: *Bring me luck, bring me wealth, and bring me the things which will bring comfort.*

Magical spells: Take a few sprigs of the herb (fresh is better but dried will work) and put it in your wallet to attract money. If you are a store owner, plant it in the front of your business to both attract shoppers and keep out people who mean to cause you harm.

Jasmine (*Jasminum officinale*)

Common names: True jasmine, summer jasmine, moonlight on the grove, poet's jasmine, and jessamine

Description: Jasmine grows up to 20 feet tall on slender stems with clinging tendrils that must be supported by a trellis or arbor. The leaves grow opposite one another on the stem, are dark green in color, and are pinnate shaped. The very fragrant whitish-yellow flowers have a tubular base that grows off new shoots, and the flowers, each of which has five petals, grow in clusters. The berry is small, dark purple, and has one small seed.

Parts used: Flowers, leaves, and roots

Cautions: None known

Folklore and history: Worshippers of Vishnu have been stringing flowers and offering them during his festivals since approximately the twelfth century. These necklaces are also given to esteemed guests at events. It is said that the jasmine flower represents the goddess as maiden, intoxicating and beautiful to behold but impossible to capture and keep, due to the fleeting nature of the flower's scent once picked. The flowers are so delicate that in order to make the oil, they must be picked in the morning, just as the dew dries, and placed between two glass panes with a layer of oil as a carrier in order to pull out the scent (the name for this process is enfleurage). The flowers are replaced in this oil mixture daily until the fat has been saturated with the scent of the flowers.

Spiritual uses: Attraction spells for love, beauty, and money; it should be noted, however, that jasmine attracts deeper types of love, inner beauty, and long-term financial strength. I have used it during weddings to ensure long-lasting marriages, and I have also used jasmine to help people see the inner beauty in themselves and others. It is a spiritual herb of the highest order, and it can help people connect with the deepest aspects of what they are trying to obtain. I make special incense for Pagan weddings that has jasmine, lavender, and rose petals in it. I give this incense to the couples as a gift to burn once a month during the full moon to remind each other of the specialness of their relationship. I also make aphrodisiac mead with jasmine flowers as one of the ingredients. I give this to newly married couples to drink on their first anniversary to solidify their marriage. Using jasmine essential oil is very expensive, but if worn, it can intoxicate a potential partner and draw them to you.

Spiritual anecdote: I once officiated a wedding that was very stressful for the bride and groom. It was so stressful that they called the wedding off twice to reconsider. I talked to them about what they really wanted, which was to love each other forever and to get the wedding stress over with. I made them both a tea to help them relax and keep the greater goal of loving one another forever in mind. The beverage contained a base of oolong tea, jasmine flowers, and mimosa flowers. This tea allowed them to have the energy to get through the wedding planning process and relax, added joy into their lives, and helped them get to the wedding day. I gave them a big jar of the tea as a wedding present and told them to drink it when they got stressed. They have been married for more than twelve years as of this writing and are still very much in love.

Astrological association: Moon

Deities, angels, or spirit associations: Vishnu, Diana of Ephesus, and Quan Yin

Meditation: Flower of purist beauty and love, grant me what my soul needs to further my (spiritual growth or true love).

Magical spells: Take 1 cup of jasmine flowers and infuse them in 2 cups of almond oil starting at the full moon closest to the summer solstice and ending at the next full moon. Strain the flowers and use the oil to anoint candles for love or to increase spirituality. To help find a spiritual connection or true love, rub this oil over your heart chakra and in the palms of your hands daily.

Jewelweed (*Impatiens pallida* or *Impatiens capensis*)

Common names: Touch-me-not, wild balsam, balsamweed, slipperweed, silver weed, wild lady's-slipper, speckled jewels, wild celandine, and quick-in-the-hand

Description: Jewelweed is an annual plant that grows in moist soil at the edge of marshes and wet forests. It grows between 2 and 5 feet tall and blooms during late summer. The leaves are pale green and have small hairs growing on them, which makes the leaf look like it has a silver sheen when under water. The leaves are ovate in shape and have teeth that surround the edges; they grow in an alternate pattern around a thin, translucent, fluid-filled stem. The flowers are trumpet shaped, ending with either a backward spur (*Impatiens biflora*) or a downward spur (*Impatiens pallida*). The opening of the flower appears to have two lips with the lower one being larger and protruding out farther than the upper one. *Impatiens pallida* flowers are pale yellow, while the flowers of *Impatiens biflora* are orange with brown speckles. The seedpods explode as soon as they are touched, giving them the common name of touch-me-not.

Parts used: Flowers, leaves, and seedpods

Cautions: Do not ingest; it can cause stomach discomfort.

Folklore and history: Most of the folklore about this plant is Native American in nature. I learned from a Cherokee shaman that it's used as a green corn medicine during the green corn ceremony and that it's used medicinally for skin rashes, to treat poison ivy and nettle rashes, and during childbirth to assist with labor (by bathing the woman's genitals in a decoction). Many Indigenous tribes use it for skin afflictions related to exposure to poison ivy, poison oak, or poison sumac, while others, including the Ojibwe, use it (decocted) as an eye wash for sore eyes and internally for kidney disease. The Ojibwe also rub it on the head to relieve headaches and use it more as an external pain reliever.

Spiritual uses: Jewelweed is by far one of my favorite plants, and I remember the first time I saw it. I was walking in the swamp on the other side of my forest and saw its bright orange, speckled head on thin, translucent stalks. I thought it was some rare type of Minnesota orchid, and I considered myself blessed to have it growing on my property. Because I had a nice-sized patch on the edge of my forest, I got to study it and see how to use it. One of the things I noticed right away was the flower heads nodding in the wind, so I used to ask it yes/no questions, and I got pretty accurate answers when I used it as a divination tool. I also noticed that the fey love this plant. They love to sit and swing in the flower heads, and I often heard music when the fey were playing in it. I imagine the fey saw it as a brightly colored, jewellike plant that they were attracted to. I harvested some from my field to make an oil for poison ivy, and I also noticed that the oil and salve I made from the plant did two other things. First, it attracted the fey, so my spiritual group used it during fairy rituals. In addition, I noticed it was also a great filtering and blocking agent against things I didn't want, so I started using the oil to neutralize or block negative actions, attitudes, or magic. Jewelweed also has a little of the trickster element to it, so if a person is working with coyote medicine or the deity Loki, this plant might be helpful.

Spiritual anecdote: I had a friend who liked to do magic in systems he really didn't understand and messed things up. One day he called me, talking about some kind of magical trouble he had gotten himself into. To help him, I anointed some brown candles with jewelweed oil in order to neutralize the chaotic and negative energy he had brought into his life. I also had him rub down all his tools with the oil and take a bath infused with some fresh jewelweed leaves. I then suggested he make some simple offerings to his deity for a few days and see if things calmed down, which they did. I gave him some of the salve I made for poison ivy and instructed him to use it so that he could neutralize any negativity before it got out of control.

Astrological associations: Venus and Mars

Deities, angels, or spirit associations: The fey and Loki

Meditation: O jewel of the forest glade, bring me the joy of the fey this way, and let me see them and join in their play.

Magical spell: Make infused oil using 1 part fresh jewelweed leaves and 2 parts olive oil. While making it, concentrate on what you want to use it for. I use the oil either to see, communicate, and play with the fey or to neutralize negative or chaotic spiritual situations.

Juniper (*Juniperus communis*)

Common names: Guinevere, ginny, *genièvre*, gin plant, joon, juni, juno, and nip

Description: Juniper is an evergreen, coniferous shrub or small tree occurring throughout the world that grows up to 6 feet tall; it can be either prostrate or erect. Its preferred location is undergrowth in mixed, open forests. As its botanical name, *communis*, suggests, juniper often occurs in groups. The bark is chocolate brown tinged with red. The leaves, 1 to 1½ inches long, are needlelike and stalkless, occurring in whorls of three. They are pale green below and dark, shiny green on the other three sides. The male plant bears a cone ¾ inch long, and the female develops a much smaller one. The fruit, which is about ½ inch in diameter, appears on the female plant. Initially green, it turns purplish black with a grayish bloom in the second and third years and has a triangular indentation at the apex. Flowering takes place in April and May, and the fruits ripen in September and October of the following year.

Parts used: Leaves and berries

Cautions: Juniper berries can be over stimulating to the kidneys; do not use for long periods of time internally or if someone has kidney disease.

Folklore and history: According to M. Grieve, during the Renaissance juniper was used in art to represent chastity, and you can often see it in artwork as a sprig of a bush or a tree. From the medieval period up to about 1850, it was documented that in Europe juniper branches were burned in large bonfires in the centers of fields and cattle were walked through the smoke to protect the livestock from harm. There is a tree spirit in Germany called Frau Wachholder, who was invoked to make thieves return stolen goods. This was done by taking two juniper branches and crossing one over the other while saying the Lord's Prayer. The cross was then hung outside the door to cause the thieves to return the stolen objects. Saint Juniper, who was one of the original followers of Saint Francis of Assisi, is sometimes called the Saint of Comedy; his feast day is January 29, and juniper is burnt in honor of him. In *Sea Priestess* by Dion Fortune, the heroine burns juniper, sandalwood, and myrrh as an offering to the goddess on the beach.

Spiritual uses: Attracting love, retrieving stolen items, health, and purification; put it in feast night meat to flavor it and use some of the flavored meat as an offering.

Spiritual anecdote: I know a woman who had some of her prized spiritual jewelry stolen at an open sabbat at her house. She thought she knew who did it, so she made a large bonfire in the backyard and burned juniper branches and myrrh as an offering to Frau Wachholder to help her get her stolen jewelry back. The person who had taken it must have had a bit of remorse, and at the next open sabbat, the jewelry was returned to its rightful owner without anyone ever knowing who really took it.

Astrological associations: Sun and Jupiter

Deities, angels, or spirit associations: Frau Wachholder, Sekhmet, Zeus, and Hera

Meditations: For love, say: *O lover, come to me to bring me happiness and love.*

For protection, use it as an herbal wand, and while cleaning the area, think: *O herb so pure and chaste, clean me and my house so that it is a sacred space.*

Magical spell: For health, take two juniper branches and tie them together with a green thread while visualizing the healing that needs to take place. Put this charm in the afflicted person's bedroom in a place they can see it.

Kava (*Piper methysticum*)

Common names: Kava kava, kava kava awa, and ava

Description: Kava is a vining plant that grows in warm climates. The part used is the roots, and they can grow 2 feet down and out from the center. The stalks grow from nodes on the roots, and each stalk can grow up to 6½ feet. Once the stalks achieve that length, the plant starts thickening up like a bush. The stalks are medium green and have nodes on them, and from these nodes the alternating leaves and rootlets emerge. The heart-shaped leaves are medium to dark green in color and have a crinkly texture with a smooth edge. Kava has both female and male plants, and the males produce most of the flowers. A kava flower is a single spike that grows up to 6 inches long. When the flower matures, it turns orange. Kava does not produce seeds. Instead, it reproduces solely through its spreading roots.

Parts used: Roots

Cautions: Do not drive or work heavy machinery after using kava; do not take with antidepressants or Parkinson's medications or mix with alcohol. It may make some people irritated, anxious, or paranoid.

Folklore and history: Kava is a Polynesian herb, and traditionally it was collected by the Indigenous women of the islands for rituals. The women would chew the root and spit it out into a large bowl. Water was added to the root and saliva mixture, and it was then drunk. Some Polynesian tribes did not chew the root first and simply soaked the root in water before they added more water and drank it. Traditionally, the drinking of this beverage is followed by a huge feast to help the beverage work better because the fat in the meal makes the kava root last longer.

Spiritual uses: Trance induction, hypnosis, astral travel, and sexual rites; I have used kava to help people get into a state of trance.

Spiritual anecdote: I've made strong tisane with kava and vervain to serve to participants before astral travel workings, and it has helped even those who've had the hardest time with astral travel. On one of these trance inductions, one of the more sensitive participants felt the ocean around her and found herself in a boat, rowing with twelve men who said that they would take her to the place she needed to go. She then traveled to an island where she found the spiritual flower she needed to perform some magic. She thought she was in Fiji but couldn't be sure. When we looked up the flower online, we found out that it was an orchid that only grows on three islands, one of which is Fiji.

Astrological association: Pluto

Deities, angels, or spirit associations: Pele and Lono

Meditation: *As deep as your roots penetrate the earth and as your tendrils reach for the sky, help me bridge the worlds and learn its secrets.*

Magical spell: Mix equal parts kava and blue vervain with 2 cups of hot water and steep for thirty minutes. Drink 1 cup prior to any ritual or astral travel to assist the journey.

Lady's Mantle (*Alchemilla vulgaris*)

Common names: Lion's foot, bear's foot, nine hooks, stellaria, and wound-wort

Description: A perennial, this plant rises from a single stalk, grows up to 2 feet tall, and has bright green leaves that are shaped like a kidney or a cape with finely toothed margins and have veins that come from where the stem attaches in the center, giving it a ruffled appearance. The small flowers bloom from July to August, are a greenish yellow, and come from multiple stems emerging from the roots.

Parts used: Leaves

Cautions: None known

Folklore and history: This plant was used so much to stanch bleeding throughout history that a common name for it became woundwort. All parts of the plant, including the roots, were used to this end. The roots, which were said to be the strongest protection against internal bleeding, were decocted and given to German soldiers as late as the twentieth century. The dew that collects on the leaves is sometimes referred to as "fairy honeydew," and it is considered an intoxicating beverage for the fey folk. It is also said that if you collect the dew off its leaves at dawn every day, you will never grow old. This herb was used by alchemists as a catalyst to change one substance into another.

Spiritual uses: This herb can be used for love magic, but I use it most in protective magic, and it works on all levels. It protects against physical, mental, and spiritual harm, especially when carried. It is also a beautification and youth-restoring herb.

Spiritual anecdote: I once had a client who was involved in a nasty situation with a negative magical person who was lying to anyone who would listen. This person went as far as to call his work, trying to get him fired, and his family to harass them. I felt that my client needed not only physical protection but mental and spiritual protection as well. To assist, I made him a protective bag that contained a small round mirror (to reflect the negativity back), lady's mantle, jet, and rutilated quartz. Within a week, the person who was doing all this harm was pulled over for a traffic violation and was sent to jail because they had a warrant out for their arrest. My client never heard from them again.

Astrological associations: Mars and Venus

Deities, angels, or spirit associations: Gaia and Artemis

Meditation: I call ye to my aid, plant of protection. Lay your cloak around me, covering me with the protection of the goddess.

Magical spells: I use it in protection magic mostly, but I also collect the dew off the leaves, whenever I remember, to keep looking young. One of the best ways to use it for protection is to put it into a gris-gris bag along with other protective herbs and have the person carry it.

Lavender (*Lavandula angustifolia*)

Common names: English lavender, true lavender, and narrow-leaf lavender

Description: Lavender is a shrubby, woody perennial bush that grows up to 3 feet tall and 2 feet wide. On each stem grows the evergreen, lance-shaped, 2½-inch-long, grayish-green leaves that develop in opposite pairs up the stem. The flowers grow at the ends of long, stiff spikes that come from the ground. The purple, double-lipped flowers that grow in clusters at the terminal ends of the stems are small and tubular at the base. All parts of the plant are highly aromatic.

Parts used: Flowers

Cautions: Inhaling too much of the essential oil or drinking too much of it as an herbal tea can cause headaches.

Folklore and history: Lavender has a large history of use as a nervine, relieving everything from headaches to epilepsy throughout the world. It was taken as an herbal tea or steeped in wine for medicinal use and even used on animals to avoid lice and illness. The Romans placed a great value on it because, as was said in *A Modern Herbal* by M. Grieve, the Romans thought that "the asp, a dangerous kind of viper, made lavender its habitual place of abode, so it had to be approached with great caution." In the Middle Ages, lavender was put on the midsummer bonfires as an offering, and it had a reputation as an herb to promote love. The Victorians revived an old custom of weaving lavender into wands to attract love and used to stuff pillows with it to help promote sweet dreams.

Spiritual uses: Dried lavender flowers can be used in incense, baths, oils, or gris-gris bags for love, health, snake magic, peace, and divination. Fresh or dried lavender stalks with flowers on them can be woven while infusing them with magical workings. I keep a vase of dried lavender flowers on stalks by my computer at work to keep my office peaceful.

Spiritual anecdote: I have used lavender for so many things, but my favorite use for the herb is dispelling negativity and restoring peace. I once had a set of friends who were dating. The only problem was that they fought all the time and were constantly bickering. So, before they would come over to my peace-filled sanctuary, I would put dried lavender and table salt in a bowl and place it by the front door. This stopped their fighting the minute they entered my house and for about an hour after they left. I have recommended this method to many of my clients to reduce general negativity and to increase peace in their homes and workspaces, telling them to keep a bowl of the mixture out constantly and to replace it at each full moon for optimal strength.

Astrological association: Mercury

Deities, angels, or spirit associations: Minoan Snake Goddess, Hestia, Aphrodite, and Hygeia

Meditation: *Herb so pure and chaste, grant me the (peace, love, or healing) I need to get me through the day and help me live with the (peace, love, or healing) I need to make me whole.*

Magical spell: Make a simple incense with 1 part lavender flowers, 1 part red rose petals, and ½ part cinnamon and burn it to strengthen love that is already there. This incense also helps bring peace and calm in times of extreme stress.

Lemon Balm (*Melissa officinalis*)

Common names: Melissa, sweet Melissa, lemon mint, bee balm, and sweet balm

Description: Lemon balm grows up to 3 feet tall and has a relatively shallow root system for the size of the plant. The dark green, gently toothed leaves grow up to 3 inches long in opposite pairs up the stem. They have a rough texture that, when rubbed, emit a strong green-lemon scent.

The flowers grow between the leaf sets at the top of the plant in July or August. They are small, white, and grow around the stem in a whorl. The seeds are small, round, and dark brown.

Parts used: Leaves

Cautions: May intensify the effects of pain medicine or valerian root

Folklore and history: Lemon balm was used by Paracelsus to restore the nerves after a traumatic event, and according to Dioscorides, "The leaves steeped in wine were used to cure the scorpion stings and the bites of mad dogs." Culpeper says that "it causes the mind and the heart to become merry and revives the heart, faintings and swoonings." Lemon balm was once used in the worship of Diana in her temples. Lemon balm is the key ingredient in Carmelite water, which is an alcoholic extraction of twenty-three herbs and spices created by the Discalced Carmelite nuns in 1611. Carmelite water was created to help with health conditions, but it was also worn by the Queen of France, who said that it made her look younger.

Spiritual uses: Healing, divination, youth promotion, or love magic; lemon balm can also be used to help people ground, especially those who are psychic and hearing voices or having uncontrollable visions from the spirit world. In such situations, I use lemon balm to make an herbal tea and do some simple grounding/energy exercises with the person while burning some purification incense. This seems to work best when the person drinks the tea at least twice a day for a week. To use lemon balm to help with divination, you can drink a cup of the tea while meditating on a question or before using tarot cards to help you get an answer. It can also help you maintain a youthful appearance, and it can be taken daily as an herbal tea or tincture to promote youth. This works best to maintain youth rather than to recapture it, but it does work to help make people look and feel a little younger.

Spiritual anecdote: I had a Native American client who had several medical issues. She had a history of slow-healing wounds and anxiety related to her living situation. She also kept making contracts with God that she felt he was ignoring. I gave her tinctures but also made her a small bag in red flannel. I then put lemon balm, lavender, sandalwood, and rosemary in bag; I added the lemon balm for healing, lavender to relieve anxiety and to help her stay calm and uplifted on rough days, sandalwood to help her reconnect with her spiritual side and her ancestors (her grandfather had been a well-respected shaman when he was alive), and rosemary to help her remember who she was on a personal and spiritual level—as well as on a tribal level.

Astrological association: Jupiter

Deity, angel, or spirit association: Diana

Meditation: Herb of sunshine bright, help me heal this wound a'right. Use your green to weave it tight; fill it with your healing might!

Magical spells: To promote health, place lemon balm in a bag with other herbs. To promote youth, you can drink it daily as an herbal tea mixed with blue vervain. You can also put the beverage in a spray bottle and spray it on daily to attract love or help maintain youth.

Lotus, Sacred (*Nelumbo nucifera*)

Common names: Chinese arrowroot, Chinese water lily, Indian lotus, Eastern lotus, East Indian lotus, Egyptian sacred bean, *padma*, and water bean

Description: The sacred lotus is an aquatic plant that has rhizomes deep in the earth. The rhizomes are long and white and can extend as far as 3 feet deep. The stems rise up from the roots, are medium green in color, and each produce a flower or leaves at the top. The leaves are round, medium green, and either cup or funnel shaped with ruffled edges. The stems grow up to 6 feet above the water. The flowers produced, which can grow up to 10 inches wide, have twelve to thirty pink, lavender, or white petals with one hundred to four hundred bright yellow stamens around each seedpod. The seedpod is round, light yellow, and has multiple holes in it called carpels, which is where the seeds mature. The seeds are large and creamy white.

Parts used: Flower, leaves, and seeds

Cautions: None known

Folklore and history: The lotus flower has a long spiritual and medicinal history that goes back to before there were written records. In Buddhism and Hinduism, the sacred lotus flower has many spiritual associations that are woven into religious philosophy. In Hinduism the sacred lotus is a symbol of divinity, life, fertility, and beauty. The unfolding of the petals represents the soul expanding as it attains enlightenment, and it's believed that the spirit of the sacred lotus is a part of each human's soul, which guides us toward the Divine. In Buddhism the sacred lotus represents the journey through life. From the dirt, the plant grows through the water just so its flowers can reach the sun. The blossoming of the flower symbolizes spiritual illumination, divinity, wisdom, and spiritual enlightenment. The Egyptians also used lotus as part of their sacred and medicinal rituals. You can see it in hieroglyphics and Egyptian art. Even though the lotus pictured in early Egyptian art may be blue lotus, by the late periods, the sacred lotus was also being used. All parts of the lotus plant are edible and can be found in many Asian grocery stores.

Spiritual uses: Fertility, wisdom, spiritual enlightenment, and transformation; it can also be used as a relaxant or mild hypnotic.

Spiritual anecdote: I used to work at an herb store in Minneapolis, and I often had people coming in asking for lotus petals, which they would smoke in order to get a mild euphoria. I had a friend who was a swami, and I asked him about this practice. He explained how sacred the flower is and how it can bring a person closer to the Divine. I asked him about smoking the petals, and he said that those who smoked the flower were only trying to attain enlightenment without doing the work. By taking a shortcut, they would end up further from cosmic enlightenment and continue their suffering. After that conversation, I tried to talk people into using different herbs for smokables.

Astrological association: Sun

Deities, angels, or spirit associations: Vishnu, Brahma, Kubera, Lakshmi, Saraswati, Isis, Horus, and Manipadmi

Meditation: To help release you or someone from negativity, greed, or lust, say *om mani padme hum* three times. It means "the jewel is in the center of the lotus."

Magical spell: Infuse sacred lotus leaves in almond oil until the scent of the lotus is in the oil. Store the oil and wear it when meditating or doing trance work to help bring you closer to the Divine.

Mandrake (*Mandragora officinarum*)

Common names: Gallow's root, mandragora, manroot, Satan's apple, liferoot, herb of Circe, and sorcerer's root

Description: Mandrake has a large, dark brown root that grows 3 to 4 feet in length. It can be a single or double tap root. The leaves are dark green, grow directly from the crown of the root, and can reach up to 1 foot long. The leaves are lance shaped with deep veins and a slightly fetid odor. The bell-shaped flowers grow on a stalk coming from the center of the crown. They are approximately 1 inch long, white, and tinged with purple. They have a mildly crinkly appearance. These flowers are followed by a smooth, round, golden-yellow fruit, the size of a small apple.

Parts used: Roots and leaves

Caution: Plant is toxic when ingested in large amounts; make sure you are getting *Mandragora officinarum* when doing magic. Other plants (usually mayapple) are often substituted for this root because of its rarity.

Folklore and history: A lot of European folklore has been documented about this plant. According to Gerard, it was said that the root should only be pulled out of the ground by a mad dog because it would drive a person mad if they tried to pull it out themselves. Gerard also said that it grew under the gallows; it was said that the blood from the criminals made it grow.

In *Zalmoxis, the Vanishing God*, author Mircea Eliade discusses how mandrake root was harvested in Romania by several old wisewomen who'd go out at dawn to collect the plant. He said that they used it for magic ideally between Easter and early June and that they had a specific way to harvest the roots. The women would bring a feast and an offering to the mandrake plant. They would then dig up the root and set out the feast around it. As the women ate, they would talk about what the root was to be used for. Once they finished eating, a coin, some sugar, and some wine were poured into the hole the mandrake was pulled from as an offering. If the magical act needed was for a girl to get a husband, the girl would go out to the plant with a wisewoman, and, after feasting, the two would grasp hands and dance naked around the root while chanting:

Mandragora, good plant
Marry me after a month.
For if you can't marry me
I'll eat what fasting forbids,
For if you don't bring him to me,
I'll eat everything that fasting forbids.

The most important information I found in the lore from Romania is that the mandrake should be collected by women and that they should be joyful when collecting and carrying the plant. If negative thoughts are present or negative things are done, the magic from the plant will dissipate.

Spiritual uses: In most of Europe, the plant was used primarily for love or wealth, but it has also been used for everything from promoting fertility to becoming more beautiful. In Romania the herb was used to make women beautiful, promote fertility, arrange a marriage, or make business more successful. It was also used against enemies and against other women when trying to get a man.

Spiritual anecdote: I have used mandrake for a fertility spell. The woman I was helping had tried everything, from magic to in vitro, and it wasn't working; this didn't seem to be an average case of infertility. I told her that if she could get a whole mandrake root, we could perform a spell. She brought me the root, and I proceeded with the first step, which involved rehydrating the root in warm water overnight. Once the root was rehydrated, I placed it under her bed, soaking it in an herb-infused wine, and told her to give it a drop of her blood every day. She was pregnant within two months. I had her then take the root, rinse it off, put it in a Mason jar, and cover it with brandy. I instructed her to take three drops of this brandy using an eye dropper every week throughout her pregnancy. This small amount of mandrake tincture was to make sure the magic that caused the pregnancy stayed in her system. I had her keep the tincture, and she used it to get pregnant with her second and third child. Those pregnancies happened easily and now she has three beautiful—and slightly magically inclined—children.

Astrological association: Saturn

Deities, angels, or spirit associations: Bendis, Diana, Hecate, and Hathor

Meditation: Imagine how obtaining something you desire will fill you with joy. Focus that energy toward the plant and say: *O Mandrake, giver of all* (insert your desire), *help me attain my desire. I need your help to get me* (insert what you need) *so that I may be happy and fulfilled.*

Magical spell: To have mandrake bring you what you desire, say the plant's meditation while laying out a feast for you and the plant. Make sure to have wine, a coin, and bread or sugar to give as an offering. Then eat and make merry with the plant. Think only joy-filled thoughts while you are doing your magical workings.

Mastic (*Pistacia lentiscus*)

Common names: Tears of Chios, Indian mastic, Turkish mastic, and megilp

Description: Mastic is a large, bush-like tree that grows up to 20 feet tall and 12 feet wide. The bark is light gray to brown in color and deeply grooved. The main trunk comes out of the ground, and the branches spread low and wide. The leaves are leathery and olive green. They grow alternately up the branches. The flowers are small and pale green with five petals and pink stamens that grow in clusters. The berries are red black in color, and each berry has one medium-sized, light brown seed with a green seed coat.

Parts used: Resin

Cautions: None known

Folklore and history: According to Gerard's *Herbal*, resin from mastic trees has been used for more than 2,500 years as a medicine, food additive, and ritual aid. As medicine it was used to treat skin wounds and mouth issues; in ritual it was used as incense or in anointing oil. Mastic was often used in ritual or celebration cakes, meals, and wine. Mastic was so popular during the Ottoman Empire that it was worth its weight in gold. It is still used today in Christian rituals in a holy anointing oil called chrism or myron, which contains several resins, including frankincense and myrrh. It is very similar to a purification oil applied to the Oracles of Delphi. According to Budge's *Egyptian Magic*, the Egyptians referred to mastic as "the fragrance that pleases the gods." It was used as an offering to the Greek and Egyptian gods and was a large part of their rituals.

Spiritual uses: Attracting spirits, spirit communication, increasing the power of other spells, improving psychic abilities, and improving communication; mastic is a great addition to incense that is used specifically for calling spirits.

Spiritual anecdote: I had a friend who practiced ceremonial magic. We had a lot of good conversations about how to attract and control the spirits that came to visit, and my friend told me about attracting certain beings to help him win the lottery. Now, I probably don't have to tell you that this never worked because sometimes the spirits one attracts are really out to play tricks or cause damage. I made my friend a blend of incense that included mastic and sweetgrass. (In many Native American traditions, sweetgrass is often used to call sweet spirits into a space once the area is purified.) This incense blend did improve his ability to call nicer spirits to his rituals, but he still didn't win the lottery.

Astrological association: Sun

Deities, angels, or spirit associations: Apollo, Athena, Hermes, Thoth, and Isis

Meditation: Resin of communication and divination, give me clear sight into the future and help me find the answers I need.

Magical spell: Take one part mastic, one part frankincense, and one part clary sage leaves and mix them together. Burn the mix on charcoal before and during divination; this mix works especially well if used when gazing into crystal balls, mirrors, or scrying bowls.

Mistletoe (*Viscum album*)

Common names: Birdlime mistletoe, European mistletoe, herb de la croix, mystyldene, and lignum crucis

Description: Mistletoe is an evergreen, hemiparasitic plant that grows in the branches of trees in round bushes that can reach up to 5 feet in diameter. The root of the mature plant can be thick and woody, but the stems that come from it are thin, light yellowish green, and vining in nature. The 1-to-3-inch-long, dark green leaves grow off the stem in pairs, are tongue shaped, and have smooth edges. The flower clusters grow in the middle of the V-shaped intersections between the branches and leaf stems. The flowers are small, yellow, and grow in groups of three to six. The berries are small, white, and slightly translucent, also growing in clusters of three to six. Each berry has a small, black seed. The plant is spread by birds, and when the sticky berries come in contact with a tree's bark, they send out thin tendrils that attach to the bark and start drawing nutrients from the tree.

Parts used: Leaves and berries

Cautions: Do not eat or burn the berries, as they are poisonous; the leaves should be eaten in moderation, as they affect heart functions. If you are on blood pressure medicine, do not ingest without consulting your physician. Use the natural, uncolored plant; the mistletoe often found during the holidays is dyed dark green and treated with preservatives, which may be toxic.

Folklore and history: In his book *Natural History*, Pliny the Elder describes the harvesting of mistletoe by Druids who, on the sixth day of the moon, prepared a ritual sacrifice and feast beneath a sacred oak tree that contained mistletoe. The ritual called for bringing two white bulls, whose horns were bound together, while a priest in white climbed the tree to cut down the mistletoe with a gold sickle, which then fell onto a white cloth at the base of the tree. The bulls were then sacrificed to the gods as ritual words and songs were sung. If the mistletoe missed the cloth and fell on the ground, it foretold bad omens.

There is also lore about mistletoe involving the god Balder, who was so cheerful and gracious that light came from him. He was the son of Odin and Frigg. As the story goes, both Balder and his mother had a dream that he would die, so Frigg asked all the animals and plants— except for mistletoe—to promise not to hurt Balder. Loki, hearing this, made an arrow out of mistletoe and handed it to Balder's blind brother to throw at him. The arrow killed Balder, but because he was so loved by the gods, the underworld returned him to life.

Spiritual uses: Rebirth, resurrection, love, fertility, protection against lightning, and opening locked physical and spiritual doors/items

Spiritual anecdote: I live in Florida, the state that has the highest number of lightning strikes in the country, so I have sprigs of yarrow and mistletoe in my windows to prevent lightning from hitting my house. I wrap each sprig in red thread and hang them in my windows. I replace them yearly to make sure the magic is strong.

Astrological association: Jupiter

Deities, angels, or spirit associations: Aphrodite, Balder, Odin, and Frigg

Meditation: Herb so small but powerful, guide me and help me open doors so that I can obtain (insert what you wish to obtain).

Magical spell: Take a sprig of mistletoe and place it in a white cloth bag along with agrimony to open closed doors and help you obtain all of your desires. Say the plant's meditation three times while concentrating on your goal. After that, carry the cloth bag with you wherever you go.

Mugwort (*Artemisia vulgaris*)

Common names: Artemis herb, felon herb, naughty man, sailor's-tobacco, Saint John's plant, and *Cingulum Sancti Johannis*

Description: Mugwort lives in partly sunny waysides and forest clearings. It is a tall-growing plant (reaching up to 6 feet) with purple-tinted, square stems. The leaves are smooth and deeply serrated, resembling a wild geranium or motherwort plant. The leaves are a darker shade of green on the top and a white, soft down on the bottom. The leaves have a green scent upon rubbing. The flowers are creamy white, oval, and end on a pinnacle. The seeds are very small and dark brown. The plant spreads by seeds and underground runners.

Parts used: Leaves

Cautions: None known

Folklore and history: It is said in Gerard's book *The Herbal* that mugwort derived its name from its use in beer production, as it was used before the introduction of hops. It was also written in that text that John the Baptist wore a girdle of mugwort in the wilderness to protect him from wild beasts.

The downy leaves have been used in the Chinese healing art of moxibustion for thousands of years. The downy hairs of the plant are separated from the leaf, and the down is rolled into cones and burned on an acupressure point relating to the pain or disease.

Mugwort is believed to protect the traveler from negative energy, sunstroke, harm from wild beasts, and evil spirits. A crown made from mugwort was worn on Saint John's eve to protect the wearer from evil possession, and it was written that if mugwort was gathered on Saint John's day, it would protect against diseases and misfortunes. It was also written in Gerard's *Herbal* that mugwort and vinegar were antidotes to henbane and sea-fish poisoning.

Spiritual uses: Psychic powers, prophetic dreaming, healing, astral projection, purification, and increasing magical strength; it can help to open the third eye to assist with divination and scrying. Mugwort works well to help the user have vivid, prophetic dreams. When used for incense, the leaf produces a slight sage-like smell, burns for a long time, and is a powerful purifier and trance enhancer.

Spiritual anecdote: As an herbalist, I see a lot of clients who sometimes need spiritual as well as medical healing. One of these times was when I saw a Native American woman who had managed to anger her tribal elders, including a powerful shaman. When she came to me for a medicinal consult, she mentioned that she also had a long run of bad luck in her life. I saw a small spiritual axe in her back with my third eye. I asked her why I was seeing this. She then started crying, telling me the whole story of how she and her family were banned from the tribe and how the tribe had cursed her for her husband's actions twenty years ago. To remove the axe, I took her into my ritual room, cast a circle, and proceeded to take the tomahawk out of her back. As I pulled it out, I saw this black substance ooze from the spiritual wound, so I grabbed the mugwort I had taken out to burn for incense and pressed it against the wound until I stopped seeing the substance come out. Even though I saw the tomahawk and wound with my third eye, the spirit of the physical herb helped heal the wound. (Mugwort is one of those herbs that easily crosses the spiritual border to get work done on the other side.) The woman was so thankful, and as of her last report, her luck had changed. She found a job doing graphic design and had gotten a nice apartment in a better neighborhood.

Astrological association: Venus

Deities, angels, or spirit associations: Diana, Pan, and Bao Gu

Meditation: *Ancient seeress, plant spirit divine, help clarify my vision; help me see what is behind.*

Magical spells: Take a clean sock or pantyhose and stuff it with mugwort and lavender. Place it under your pillow for both restful and enlightening dreams.

Mix together a tisane of 1 ounce of mugwort, 1 ounce of eyebright, and 1 ounce of cinnamon. Use 1 teaspoon of the mix per 1 cup of hot water. Drink this tisane prior to doing divination or spiritual work. It will help open the third eye and make spiritual work easier.

Myrrh (*Commiphora myrrha*)

Common names: Balsamodendron myrrha, didin, didthin, myrrha, Somali myrrh, mur, and karam

Description: The myrrh tree grows up to 13 feet tall. The trunk is grayish brown and has a thin outer bark with knots that, at times, appear to peel. The branches are low growing, mostly at right angles, and thorny; each branch has a larger spike at the end of stem. One to three leaves grow from each node along the branches. They are small, greenish yellow, and grow in a pinnate pattern. The small flowers, which grow at the base of the leaf petioles, or stems, are yellowish green with three petals and bright yellow stamens. The fruit hangs directly from the stem. It is disk shaped and initially green but turns a light maroon color when ripe.

Parts used: Resin

Cautions: None known

Folklore and history: In Greek mythology, Aphrodite cursed Myrrha with an insatiable lust for her father because Myrrha's mother bragged that Myrrha was more beautiful than the goddess. Myrrha tricked her father into having sex with her, and once he found out what happened, he tried to kill her. Myrrha ran for nine months until the gods took pity on her and turned her into a myrrh tree. Once she was a tree, she gave birth to

Adonis, who was the mortal lover of both Aphrodite and Persephone. The resin from the myrrh tree was said to be the tears of Myrrha.

Myrrh has been used for centuries as medicine, as an embalming agent, and for religious purposes. One of the first written uses of myrrh was found on the walls of the Deir el-Bahri Temple. The walls tell the story of Queen Hatshepsut's great trip to Punt and have images of barges full of cassia, myrrh resin, and live frankincense trees traveling back to Egypt with her. According to Plutarch, a Greek philosopher, the Egyptians burned incense three times a day. In the morning, as the sun rose, they burned frankincense; at noon, they burned myrrh; and when the sun set, they burned kyphi. Myrrh was a large part of the Egyptian embalming process and has been found in tombs as offerings for rulers to take with them to the underworld.

Spiritual uses: Purification, protection, fertility, lust, rebirth, removing hexes and curses, and connecting oneself with the Divine

Spiritual anecdote: Once a member of my spiritual group had been experiencing a series of tragedies that included the death of a family member, being diagnosed with diabetes, and losing the job that he had for more than a decade. Our group did some work to figure out what was causing this streak of misfortune so that we could help him with it, and one of the items that kept coming up as one of his protectors was myrrh resin. I happened to have a pound of it on hand, so I gave him a half pound and split the other half among the group. We did a curse removal spell that evening using straight myrrh as our incense, and then we decided that we would each burn some incense every night for the next seven days with the intention to break whatever curse was on him. After ten days, at the next full moon, he received news from his factory that he was being called back to work. The machine that had been brought in to replace him kept breaking down, and they had to meet a deadline. They ended up teaching him to run the machine and keep it running, giving him a higher wage, and his luck seemed to get better after that.

Astrological association: Sun

Deities, angels, or spirit associations: Adonis, Aphrodite, Isis, Sekhmet, and Ra

Meditation: *Tears of the mother, help cleanse me and purify me so that I may be worthy of your blessing of* (insert wish).

Magical spell: Place a piece of myrrh in a red flannel or velvet bag and carry it with you. This will protect you from being cursed, and it can also be used to increase fertility.

Nettle (*Urtica dioica*)

Common names: Stinging nettle and common nettle

Description: Nettles grow up to 6 feet tall, often on the edge of rivers and other wet areas. The plant has two layers of roots, the topmost layer being rhizomatic in nature. This first layer is fine and spreads like a mat across the top layers of soil, while the second is taproot-like and grows up to 6 feet deep. Both are yellowish white in color. From this rhizome many square-shaped stems rise from the ground that are covered with stinging hairs. The leaves grow up these stems in an alternating fashion and are cordate or lance shaped with serrated edges. Both the leaves and the stems have small white hairs that sting when touched. This is because they have chemicals that induce irritation to the skin, such as formic acid, histamine, and choline. Nettle flowers are either male or female. The male flowers can be purple or yellow, while the female flowers can be green or white. The flowers develop in the axils of the upper leaves and grow off of drooping panicles.

Parts used: Leaves or aerial parts of young plants and roots

Cautions: In a few individuals, exposure to the histamine in fresh nettles can be extremely dangerous. Do not eat fresh nettles; dried or cooked nettles are completely nontoxic and may be eaten freely as a vegetable or drunk as an infusion.

Folklore and history: According to M. Grieve, nettles have been used to treat arthritic conditions since the time of the Romans; they did so by taking a nettle plant and flaying their pained joints with it. This practice can be found in many folk medicine books written in the Americas as a way to treat arthritis up until the 1950s. Nettles have been historically used as a food, and the plant was cooked and added to soups and stews. Nettle

Day is May 1, and it is celebrated in Europe. It's lucky on Nettle Day to wrap a steamed nettle leaf with a dock leaf and eat it.

Spiritual uses: Money, health, protection, and removing curses; I prefer to make a nettle tisane and either drink or sprinkle it where it is needed.

Spiritual anecdote: I usually use nettle for health or money but have also used it for protection, and I remember one client who needed the herb for all three. This client was a vegetarian who needed more iron in her diet, so I gave her a nettle tisane to help with some of her mineral deficiencies. She also told me that she was having money issues because her ex-husband wasn't paying child support or alimony; he was also harassing her. After hearing this, I told her to light a green candle and concentrate on what she wanted to happen every day for a week. I also had her sprinkle a bit of her daily tisane on her wallet and on a picture of her children while the candle was lit. Her case against her ex-husband came to a judge a month earlier than it was supposed to; the judge granted her back child support, and a penalty was to be garnished from her ex-husband's wages effective immediately. He also, within a month of the spell, got a job several states away, so he could not harass her in person anymore.

Astrological association: Mars

Deities, angels, or spirit associations: Thor, Hecate, and Sekhmet

Meditation: *Nettle, strong warrior of the herbs, protect me in my time of need. Shield me from harm, returning blows sent to me back manyfold.*

Magical spells: For health, make a nettle tisane, and chant over it three times, saying, "Nettle, strong and pure, help me and create a cure." Then drink the tea.

For protection, say the plant's meditation while taking a cup of tisane and asperging it in a clockwise pattern around whatever it is you want to protect.

Nightshade, Deadly (*Atropa belladonna*) and Nightshade, Black (*Solanum nigrum*)

Common names: Belladonna, Devil's cherries, Devil's herb, naughty man's cherries, and dwale

Description: Belladonna, or deadly nightshade (*Atropa belladonna*), is a perennial plant that grows to be 3 to 4 feet tall in the northern parts of the United States and Europe. It has medium green leaves that are smooth yet soft to the touch due to very fine hairs; they grow anywhere from 1 to 4 inches in length and are oval in shape. When the fresh leaves are crushed, they emit an unpleasant, slightly pungent scent. The flowers, which appear in July, are a dingy purple in color and tinged with green around their base. The mature berry is black and shiny. When you see the berry on the plant, it looks like a black crystal ball resting on a green, five-pointed pillow.

Black nightshade (*Solanum nigrum*) is a bush-like, short-lived perennial that only grows to be about 2 feet tall, blooming in midsummer. The flowers, which are the main way to distinguish this plant, are small and white with bright yellow stamens. The flowers droop down in between the leaf sets. The leaves are dull green, have a pungent odor, and are rounded and lace shaped. The berries, when immature, are green, but when they ripen, they turn black and shiny.

Parts used: Leaves, berries, and roots

Cautions: Both varieties of nightshade are toxic and should not be taken internally at any time; nightshade can cause seizures and death when used internally. Do not use in combination with any other medications.

Folklore and history: There are many legends and myths about nightshade, including ones where witches would fly on the stems of this plant to the sabbat. It also has a long history of being used as a medicine. Belladonna is the nightshade often referred to in the older texts. According to M. Grieve, belladonna was often referred to as dwale in medieval times, while in other books, it is said that dwale was referred to as a drink that contained belladonna. Seeing as belladonna was the main ingredient in dwale, I believe that it is safe to conclude that the name refers to the herb itself.

There are several possibilities for how belladonna got its name. It might have gotten the name because Italian women used the juice of the plant to dilate their eyes and make them look more beautiful; *belladonna* means "beautiful woman." Another myth about how this plant got this name was from a superstition that said the plant took the form of a lovely enchantress who was dangerous for a man to look upon.

Spiritual uses: In small amounts, nightshade leaves can been burned in incense and used for external application as flying ointment. All nightshades contain the alkaloids hyoscyamine and scopolamine; these are the chemicals responsible for hallucination and death. In deadly nightshade, or belladonna, the leaves contain 5 percent hyoscyamine, the unripe berries contain 65 percent, and the root contains 85 percent. Ripe belladonna berries contain the chemical known as atropine, which is a cardiac stimulant used to restart the heart if it stops beating. Using the different forms of the nightshade for magical workings can be done, but extreme caution should be taken. The fresh plants are at their most toxic; dried ones are a little safer. I recommend not using this plant unless you have experience working with toxic plants.

I have used these plants in moderation when making incense for protection magic and flying ointment. In moderation belladonna can be used to assist with astral travel, drawing down the moon/sun or gods, or any other otherworldly adventure you might want to have. It does not do this by making you high—even though it may make you slightly spacey feeling. It does this by changing your consciousness so that leaving this plane is easier.

Spiritual anecdote: I make a flying ointment using this plant and several other herbs to help with astral travel, and I often save it for rituals where I need to do strong magic. One of the times my groups used it was on 9/11. Several covens convened to see what work needed to be done, and a decision was made to do work calling for justice and to help any spirits transcend from this world to the next. That night, we used the salve with nightshade in it and astral traveled to the wreckage site to see if we could help the souls who were stuck in transition.

Astrological association: Saturn

Deities, angels, or spirit associations: Atropos, Bellona, and Circe

Meditation: *Nightshade, my protector and friend, help me take flight and see in the darkness of night; show me what I need to see to assist me tonight.*

Magical spell: Take three leaves of nightshade and wrap them with a blue thread, leaving about an inch at the end unwrapped. Put the leaves in a red or orange bag along with mugwort, blue vervain, wild lettuce, and a small quartz crystal. Wear this bag when trying to channel the gods. Again, only use nightshade if you are familiar with working with deadly herbs.

Oak (*Quercus* spp.)

Common names: White oak, tanner's oak, red oak, common oak, and duir (among many others)

Description: The oak is a large, slow-growing tree indigenous to America and Europe with deep tap roots. There are many types of oak trees in this family, and each has a different bark and leaf style depending on species; most oaks can be used interchangeably for magical workings. Many oak trees have gray bark with fissures of varying depth. The leaves grow in a spiral pattern around the branches. Some oak leaves are simple, some have complex lobes, some have serrated edges, and some have smooth borders. Oak trees have both male and female flowers. The male flowers are catkins that hang down, while the female flowers are small and whitish. Because the trees have both male and female flowers, oak is considered self-pollinating. The acorns are the nut of the oak tree and are high in tannins. Each acorn has one to two seeds in it and is surrounded by a hard, leathery cover that can be green when unripe and brown or black in color when ripe. The acorn is covered with a medium brown, textured cap called a cupule, which attaches to the branch of the tree.

Parts used: Inner bark, stems, and acorns

Cautions: If you are going to eat the acorns, make sure to leach the tannins out of them, or they will make you ill.

Folklore and history: According to Pliny the Elder's writings, oak was sacred to the Greeks and Romans; the Romans dedicated it to Jupiter. Pliny also says that it was venerated by the Druids, and that every Druid gathering was held underneath an oak tree. Old folktales from the region of the Sherwood Forest say that fairies danced around the oak trees; some of the oldest trees in England are oaks in the Sherwood Forest. In Galen's book *On the Constitution of the Art of Medicine*, he recommends applying the bruised leaves to wounds to heal them. Its botanical name, *Quercus*, is derived from the Celtic *quer*, meaning "fine," and *cuez*, meaning "tree."

Spiritual uses: Protection against lightning and thieves, increasing strength, purity of heart, virtue, healing, luck, channeling energy, and grounding; acorn caps make great fairy cups on an altar. Oak wood that has been struck by lightning is excellent to make magical tools with as they will be more powerful. I really like making magical tools out of oak because it adds strength to the workings, and I once got a piece of wood from a tree that was struck by lightning. I used it to make a wand, which was quite strong. I also use the wood in protection spells against bad weather, and I have a Brigid's cross I made with oak and red thread to trap bad weather (hurricanes, tornadoes, etc.). One year we had a devastating tornado in Florida that destroyed more than fifty homes. It hit the subdivision next to us, jumped ours, and landed in the subdivision to the left of us, staying on the ground and causing millions of dollars in damage. I am not sure if it was the oak specifically, but the protective magic we did to protect our homestead from storms must have worked.

Spiritual anecdote: I once had a magical student who had a real issue sending and grounding energy. They could raise energy easily but couldn't channel or ground it, and after several broken electronics (due to energy just shooting out of their hands), I decided to teach them how to use an oak wand. Oak is especially suited to helping people not only channel and send energy, but ground it when the magic is done. After a few weeks of working from this wand, my student was successfully able to take the energy, put it into their workings, and then ground it.

Astrological association: Sun

Deities, angels, or spirit associations: The Dagda, Diana, Thor, Zeus, Indo-European thunder and sky gods, Hecate, and Pan

Meditation: *Ancient tree of wisdom and power, come to my aid in my time of need to protect me against* (insert what you need protecting from) *and assist me to stay safe.*

Magical spell: Carrying an acorn will offer protection, strength, the virtue to make the right decisions, and, of course, luck. Charm an acorn to protect you by saying the plant's chant while concentrating on it protecting you, then carry it whenever you need protection.

Olive (*Olea europaea*)

Common names: Olea, oleaster, and oliver

Description: A small evergreen tree that grows to be about 20 feet tall, olive has thin, smooth branches and gray bark. Its wood is known to be quite fragrant. The leaves are lance shaped, grow to be about 2 inches long, and are pale green on the top and silvery green on the underside. The flowers are small and white to a pale cream in color, each with four petals. The fruit, when ripe, is black, about ¾ inch long, and oval shaped. It contains a seed that is blunt along one side.

Parts used: Leaves, fruit, and bark

Cautions: None known

Folklore and history: Olive oil has long been used magically and in the worship of the old gods. From ancient Crete to ancient Rome, olive oil was used in the temples for everything from lighting the oil lamps to making offerings to the gods. Kings were anointed with the oil prior to the great festivals to honor the gods that had graced them with their harvest. Olive branches were made into crowns as symbols of benediction and purification and ritually offered to deities and powerful figures, as well as heroes after battle or the games.

Olive use has ancient roots. Fossilized remains of the olive tree's ancestor were found near Livorno, Italy, dating from twenty million years ago, although actual cultivation of the plant probably did not occur in that area until the fifth century BC.

Spiritual uses: Peace, restoring youth, creating wealth, and restoring virtue; I use olive oil quite frequently when making magical oil blends, when anointing candles prior to magical work, and as a moisturizer on the wood parts of my magical tools. It is an integral part of my magical and medicinal apothecary, and it can be an invaluable magical tool. The wood can also be used to make magical objects, such as offering bowls, runes, wands, and deity images.

Spiritual anecdote: I had a client who was half Greek. She came to me for medicinal herbal therapy, but she told me that she had been having these odd flashes of Zeus and violets. Now, if you know Greek mythology, you know that this ties into the story of one of Zeus's lovers, Io, whom he had to turn into a heifer to protect her because Hera discovered their affair and got jealous. Io tried to eat the grass, but it was to hard for her to eat. She started crying, so Zeus made Io's tears turn into violets for her to consume instead. After talking to my client some more, it turned out that she was seeing a much older man and her father did not approve. She did not think the older man was married, but he did have five children. I talked to her and suggested that perhaps the universe was sending her a message, telling her that sometimes things hidden in our conscious mind come out in dreams or as flashes in daydreams. To help, I gave her some olive tincture and suggested she make an offering to Hera and see if she could guide her. My client later found out that the man refused to pay child support for his children, and she figured she did not want to be involved with a man who did not take responsibility for his children.

Astrological association: Sun

Deities, angels, or spirit associations: Athena, Apollo, Zeus, and Hera

Meditation: *Sacred plant of the gods, grant me peace during hard times; lend me your beauty and assistance.*

Magical spell: This spell to maintain youth is quite easy. Simply infuse some dried rose petals, lavender, geranium, and immortelle flowers in the oil from full moon to full moon. Shake the container full of oil daily, saying, "Oil of the gods, please maintain my youth and beauty; help me stay young forever." Strain out the flowers and apply the oil to your face every night before bed.

Orange, Sweet (*Citrus sinensis*)

Common names: Seville orange and China orange

Description: Sweet orange is a subtropical evergreen tree with grayish-green bark that can grow up to 30 feet tall and 20 feet wide. Its leaves are ovate, 2 to 3 inches long, and dark green and glossy on top with a lighter green underneath. The small white flowers, which grow in clusters, have five thick, waxy petals and twenty stamens with large yellow anthers. The flowers appear in early spring and produce a heavy orange/vanilla fragrance. The fruit, which is actually a modified berry called a hesperidium, is round and bright orange with a rough-textured, thick skin. When opened the fruit has segments, with teardrop-shaped seeds in each segment.

Parts used: Flowers, leaves, and fruit

Cautions: None known

Folklore and history: The orange tree is originally from China and was cultivated as far back as 2500 BC. Oranges were brought along trade routes, making it to Europe in the 1500s, and the plant was brought to the Americas by the Spaniards. In Europe, young girls, sometimes as young as six or seven, would take a peeled orange rind and let it fall on the floor. Whatever initial the orange peel looked like would be the first initial of the person they would someday marry. In Italian lore, the orange tree was a symbol of fertility because of its flowers and the way an orange develops from where the center of the flower was. Oranges were also seen as a good luck charm in Italy, so orange trees were often given as wedding presents, and orange flowers decorated the bride's cake to ensure multiple children. Gerard states that the orange was the "apple" that Juno gave to Jupiter on their wedding day. In some parts of England, oranges are rolled downhill instead of eggs as a part of Easter games.

Spiritual uses: Divination, fertility, luck, money, and love; I use orange flower water a lot—for several things. I cook with it to help promote love (or even to promote friendship among enemies), and I spray it on my linens before bed to ensure a great night's sleep and for its love attributes. You can spray the flower water on areas where you want to attract love, or you can make an herbal tea using orange rind to promote love, luck, or money; fresh or dried orange rind will work for this. I have candied the flowers off my trees and put them on my friend's wedding cake to promote fertility.

Spiritual anecdote: One of my students was having an issue in her marriage and feared that her husband had a crush on one of his coworkers. To help, I had her mix rose and orange flower water together and told her to spray it on her sheets and on the couch in the living room after chanting the meditation I have listed for this herb. Her marriage got better quickly, and the two renewed their vows in Hawaii the following year.

Astrological association: Sun

Deities, angels, or spirit associations: Hera and Zeus

Meditation: *Beautiful flower of Juno, bring love to me (or back to me). Help me show the one I love how beautiful, kind, and loving I am so that they come to (or stay by) my side forever.*

Magical spell: Every year in December, I make old-fashioned pompadour balls that I give as gifts to my friends to help attract money. I take an orange and first poke a small hole in it. Then I poke whole cloves into it until it is full of cloves. I use a hair pin at the top to attach a green ribbon, roll them in orris root and cinnamon, and charge them for prosperity in the New Year. I hum while I make them, infusing them with this magic. My friends hang them up in their houses over their doors to increase the money coming into the household. This is a simple technique, and you can replicate it yourself when December comes around.

Palo Santo (*Bursera graveolens*)

Common names: Holy wood and holy stick

Description: Palo santo is a medium-sized tree that can grow up to 20 feet tall. The bark is smooth and brown with patches of gray. The main trunk is relatively short and branches grow off it in a vase-shaped pattern, meaning the branches grow at sharp angles upward. The elliptical-shaped leaves of palo santo grow opposite of each other up the stems and are dark green with deeply serrated edges. The flowers grow in panicles at the ends of the branches. They are small, round, and yellow white. The flowers produce round, green fruit, approximately ½ inch wide, with a single large, dark brown seed.

Parts used: Wood

Cautions: None known

Folklore and history: Palo santo is from the same family of trees (Burseraceae) as frankincense and myrrh, which also have aromatic wood. There is research that says the Aztecs used the wood for medicine and ritual, but it is not clear if the Aztecs had a certain ritual they used the wood for or what spiritual abilities that they thought it had. What is different about this tree is that the wood is traditionally only collected from fallen branches that have been left to age for two to three years; this aging concentrates the oils in the wood.

Spiritual uses: Purification, getting rid of evil spirits, removing negativity, and removing hexes and curses

Spiritual anecdote: Once I was cleaning a house that had been the location of several gruesome murders. The current owner loved the fact that there were ghosts there, but there was one entity that was very dark. This entity had tipped over chairs right in front of the owner, and once she tripped, fell, and broke a finger. She wanted that spirit to leave and to let the others decide if they wanted to stay. I had a discussion with her about how hard that would be and that all of the spirits in the house would probably leave. In the end, she decided to have me just do a cleaning of negative energy and teach her how to manage the negative spirit. Now, this is something I don't normally do because most mundane people can't do it and will make things worse, but she was a well-respected Pagan high priestess, so I taught her how to manage this negative spirit. One of the things I instructed her to do was cleanse with palo santo three days prior to the full moon while saying a chant. This helped her keep the negative spirit under control.

Astrological association: Jupiter

Deities, angels, or spirit associations: Mictlantecuhtli and Tezcatlipoca

Meditation: *Wood so holy, protect me against harm and negativity throughout the day.*

Magical spells: Use palo santo as an herbal wand to get rid of negativity, curses, or hexes. You can also carry a piece of palo santo wood with a red string around it to protect yourself against negativity or negative people.

Passionflower (*Passiflora incarnata*)

Common names: Passion vine, maracock, granadilla, and maypop

Description: Passionflower is a vining plant that grows in the southeastern United States, Central America, and South America. It can grow up to 30 feet long and 6 feet wide. The plant spreads by seeds and underground runners, which can become aggressive in tropical climates. The vines are woody and bright green when small, developing a brown bark when they grow thicker. They have multiple tendrils and branching stems with medium green leaves growing on them. Each leaf has three lobes, and each lobe has a deep yellow-green vein, pointed tip, and slightly toothed edges. The sweet-scented flowers are open by day and close at night. The flower is round and has five petals in a star shape around the center that are green on one side and purple on the other. There are five other pure purple petals placed in a similar fashion. Over those petals is a purple corolla attached at the center with a fine-cut, frilly edge. In the center, there is a set of five anthers and three stamens. The stamens brush the anthers when insects land on the flower, which self-pollinates the fruit. The fruit is egg shaped and green with multiple seeds and a delicious yellow pulp. The seeds are medium-sized and dark brown.

Parts used: Leaves

Cautions: Do not ingest during pregnancy; ingestion may cause drowsiness, dizziness, or nausea or increase the risk of asthma attacks in some individuals.

Folklore and history: When the Spanish missionaries came to North America in the late 1500s and saw passionflower for the first time, they thought that it resembled the crucifixion of Jesus because the anthers look like a crown of thorns. In Mexico the plant is used as a mild hypnotic in some rituals to help people meet the spirit that is causing them illness. There, it is also used to find true love, and the flower and roots can be made into a hummingbird charm. If you ever get a chance to see this plant in person,

I highly recommend checking it out. The scent is amazing, and high spiritual energy emits from the entire plant.

Spiritual uses: This plant is helpful for getting people to relax and be open in order to astral travel, do trance work, or perform chakra balancing; I use it the most to help with astral travel, especially for those who have a hard time with losing control of their spirit as it disconnects from their body. I have also used passionflower as a mild hypnotic to help get people into a trancelike state, and I've been using it for chakra balancing a lot as of late. It moves along the spine up through the top of the head to align all of the chakras (not just the main ones). Medicinally, I am finding that it works wonders with nerve pain and am curious whether it works along the physical nerve plexus to connect with the astral. This herb is useful when a calming and focusing agent is needed in a magical act. An example of this would be a win-in-court spell.

Spiritual anecdote: I had a student who had issues with astral travel. It wasn't that she couldn't do it, but once she realized that she was floating, she freaked out and her spirit jumped back in her body. She was growing frustrated because she wanted to astral travel. She also admitted that she was a control freak over everything in her life to the point that she was having issues in her personal life. Because of this, I had her drink a cup of passionflower leaf and chamomile tea every day. The dried passionflower leaf didn't have much of a flavor, but she loved the honey-like flavor of chamomile and felt very relaxed at the beginning of our astral travel meditation. Once we got to the part where she had issues in the past, she went through it and proceeded to have a good initial astral travel experience. She said that she not only felt relaxed but in a low level of trance, which helped her with astral travel. She continued to drink the tea every day to help keep her calm in her mundane life.

Astrological association: Venus

Deities, angels, or spirit associations: Apollo and Aphrodite

Meditation: Flower that travels between the worlds, assist me with my travels to the astral and beyond.

Magical spell: Combine 1 tablespoon of passionflower leaf, 1 tablespoon of vervain, and 1 tablespoon of chamomile and put the mix in a muslin tea bag. Place the tea bag in a cup, pour near-boiling water over it, and let it steep for twenty minutes. Remove the tea bag and add sweetener if desired. Drink about thirty minutes before astral travel or trance work to intensify the experience.

Patchouli (*Pogostemon patchouli*)

Common names: Pucha-pat and nilam

Description: Patchouli grows up to 3 feet tall. Its leaves have an oval shape, are medium green in color with yellow-green veins, and are fragrant when rubbed. The leaves grow alternating along a square stem and have finely serrated edges. The plant's flower spikes grow from the top of each stem and produce tiny lipped flowers. Each whitish-purple flower produces a seed that is very small and brown. The plant grows well in tropical and humid climates; it can also be grown indoors.

Parts used: Leaves

Cautions: None known

Folklore and history: Patchouli historically comes from Indonesia and Sri Lanka and was used as a medicine and insect repellent. In the seventeenth and eighteenth centuries, it was used to mask the smell of decomposing bodies at funerals. It gained popularity when people began to import silks from Asia, as the fine silks were wrapped with patchouli to preserve the cloth and protect it from insects on the long journeys.

Spiritual uses: Love, lust, money, healing, and protection

Spiritual anecdote: I had a client whose husband was unfaithful, and she wanted some magical tools to keep him faithful and sexually interested in her. She had low self-esteem, so we had a discussion on how beautiful and valuable she was and that any man would be crazy not to love her. I asked her to go see a counselor to work on her self-esteem, and I also gave her a blend of essential oils mixed in a sweet rum that I said a little prayer over. One of the main oils was patchouli, and it did help for a while—until she figured out that she could do better than him and left him after his next incident of cheating. Magic works best when it gets rid of the problem (i.e., the cheating husband).

Astrological association: Saturn

Deities, angels, or spirit associations: Aphrodite and Dionysus

Meditation: *Scented wonder, help me to align my desires with the universe as I seek you to assist me in increasing the presence of money and its pleasures in my life.*

Magical spell: To attract money, take a green flannel or velvet bag and fill it with half basil and half patchouli. Chant the plant's meditation over it and put it next to your wallet every night while you sleep. You can also put a leaf of patchouli in your wallet to help attract money to it.

Peppermint (*Mentha piperita*)

Common names: Balm mint, green mint, Our-Lady's-mint, brandy mint, and lamb mint

Description: Mentha is a perennial herb up to 2 to 4 feet tall with a green, square stem with a purple tinge. The leaves are 2 inches or more in length with fine-toothed borders. The leaves are smooth on the top but have some hairy surfaces on the under rib. The reddish-purple flowers bloom on whorled clusters in the axils of the top leaves. The entire plant has a characteristic odor due to the volatile oils in all parts of the plant.

Parts used: Aerial leaves

Cautions: None known

Folklore and history: There are at least thirty species of mint that can be used for herbal tea. Some research shows that *M. piperita* was cultivated by the Egyptians, and Pliny states that the Romans and Greeks wore crowns of peppermint at their feasts. The ancient Greeks also used two separate species of mint, but it is unknown what species they were. Mice and rats hate the smell of peppermint, and it can be used to repel rodents. The whole mint family was named after the Greek nymph Minthe who loved Pluto, the god of the underworld. When Pluto's wife found out about the nymph, she killed her. Pluto was so saddened by this that he brought her back from the underworld as a sweet-smelling plant.

Spiritual uses: Healing, purification, dispelling negativity, promoting love, and increasing psychic abilities; I use it a lot in teas and tisanes for love spells, divination, and healing. In fact, it acts like a catalyst for the other herbs and makes the whole thing stronger. Peppermint alone can be used during divination to increase psychic abilities, and it helps keep the reader from absorbing the client's energies.

Spiritual anecdote: One of my magical students had a stalker of sorts, and he refused to leave her alone. The police at the time didn't think much of it and after talking to the guy thought he was pretty harmless. So, I made her a bag with a small mirror, hematite, and some herbs, the main one being peppermint. I also had her sprinkle peppermint tea around her house and around her work (as best as she could). Well, the man stopped coming around almost immediately, and as my student started to breathe easy and stopped carrying her bag, he popped in while she was getting her morning coffee to say he would never see her again because he had fallen in love with someone else. She never saw him again.

Astrological association: Mercury

Deities, angels, or spirit associations: Michael the Archangel, Pluto, and Hecate

Meditation: *Plant so strong and sweet, come to my aid to assist me in protecting me and my loved ones from harm.*

Magical spell: To discover the first initial of your future love's name, sprinkle the herb in a 1-foot circle while concentrating on finding true love. You should be able to pick out an initial—and sometimes even a face—from the scattered leaves.

Plantain (*Plantago major*)

Common names: Cockoo's bread, Englishman's foot, snakebite weed, snakeweed, and white-man's footprint

Description: Plantain is a low-growing plant that only gets to be up to 20 inches tall, and it is not related to *Musa* × *paradisiaca* or any other banana species. When growing, the parts that first appear are the leaves, which are oval in shape and dark green in color. These leaves reach up to 9 inches long and 6 inches wide. They have deep veins, and if you tear the leaves across the ribs, you will find that the leaves have strings in them. These strings are one of the best ways to identify the plant prior to the stalks emerging. The stalks of the plant, once they emerge, also make it easy to identify; they grow from the center of the plant and look like an incense stick. The flowers that grow on the stalks are very small and purplish green. The seeds are also very small and are purple brown. Each plant produces many seeds and the best way to start some growing is to collect some of the stalks and spread the seeds in your yard at any time to encourage plant growth the following year.

Parts used: Leaves and seeds

Cautions: None known

Folklore and history: Plantain has been used as medicine since the time of the Romans, and it seemed to follow them as they went out to conquer the world. Plantain was used by many healers, including Pliny, Dioscorides, and Native Americans, who gave it its common name of white-man's footprint. Pliny states that "if it be put in a pot where many pieces of flesh are boiling, it will sodden them together," and Gerard says that it can cure the bite of a mad dog or bites from sea serpents. Members of many Native American tribes used to carry the leaf or root of this plant to avert the bite of snakes, and it was also used as a medicine to draw out the snake poison if bitten. One odd piece of lore from England is that they used to call it "mother-die" because supposedly if you brought a leaf of it into the house, your mother would die.

Spiritual uses: Healing, strength, repelling snakes, and removing poisonous curses; plantain can be used to protect and to repel danger, as well as in spells where you want to draw something away from you. I have used plantain in hex-removal spells and have also placed the herb in a magical bag in order to avoid danger. In fact, this is one of the few herbs I always carry with me in my magical and medicinal bag. Plantain can also be used as a magical plant guardian that will protect you in any situation. Just ask the spirit of the plant if it will guard and guide you, and if it says yes, you will have a powerful agent to call upon, even in the most mundane of situations.

Spiritual anecdote: I have many case studies related to the healing powers of this herb, but one I remember vividly involved a lady who had gotten bitten by a little boy everyone joked about being possessed. The mother thought nothing was wrong with her son, but she did hear him muttering oddities in a strange language. The lady developed a weird infection from this bite. In fact, she was in the hospital for two weeks and almost had to have her arm amputated because of it. I gave her a simple healing salve to put on it and also threw some plantain seeds in her yard so the plant would grow and protect her. I also dried out two stalks, made a cross from them, and charmed it to protect her. The wound healed, and the two women never spoke again.

Astrological association: Venus

Deities, angels, or spirit associations: Athena and Ares

Meditation: O great plant, so small and underappreciated, please be my plant ally and protect me from harm and keep evil far from me.

Magical spell: Take the root of plantain and carry it with you to avoid the poisons of others. The root works best if tied with red string or placed in a red bag for this purpose.

Poppy (*Papaver somniferum*)

Common names: Corn poppy, corn rose, and mawseed

Description: Poppy is an annual that can grow up to 3 feet tall. It's silver green, and the leaves come off the stem in an alternating fashion. The leaves, which are wider at the base, have a deep central vein and serrated and slightly ruffled edges. Sometimes there are stiff hairs on the central vein of the leaf. The flowers grow at the top of the stem and vary slightly in color but are often pink with a purple center or white with a dark pink center. The four petals of the flower are very delicate; just touching them can cause the petals to fall off. The flowers have a central corolla that turns into the cap of the poppy pod. The pod grows at the end of the stem and contains tiny dark brown seeds.

Parts used: Seeds

Cautions: None known

Folklore and history: According to M. Grieve, the earliest reference to using the poppy was 3400 BC. The Sumerians referred to it as *Hul Gil*, or "the Joy Plant." Sumerian tablets told of how the Sumerians collected the poppy juice from the flowers first thing in the morning. The Egyptians cultivated it as well and traded it to the Greeks, who used it as an anodyne to control pain and in ritual. It is said to be part of the Eleusinian

Mysteries and was often associated with Persephone and her descent into the underworld. Poppy seeds can be used in ritual to produce a hypnotic effect. One gram of poppy seeds has micro doses of both morphine and codeine. As little as 5 grams of poppy seeds can give a positive result on a drug screen, so it is best to avoid them in large doses. The white latex that comes from the plant is used to make some modern pain medications.

Spiritual uses: Relaxation, scrying, communication with the ancestors, and rituals to Persephone

Spiritual anecdotes: I have made my grandmother's poppy seed rolls before certain rituals where I need to go into a deep trance. The poppy seeds help as a way to relax the inhibitions that block communicating with the gods. I only make this recipe if I know that no one participating in the ritual will be going for a drug screen in the next thirty days because it is heavy on poppy seeds. I also had a student who used to eat a large lemon poppy seed muffin before every ritual because it helped her get relaxed for the work we were about to do.

Astrological association: Moon

Deities, angels, or spirit associations: Persephone, Demeter, and underworld deities

Meditation: Beautiful plant of the underworld, help me on my journey to the underworld to communicate with my loved ones who have passed through your doors.

Magical spell: Mix poppy seeds, basil, and frankincense in equal parts and burn it as incense in rituals involving underworld deities or when performing Egyptian rituals. Do not be surprised when the poppy seeds "pop" in the incense blend.

Queen of the Meadow (*Filipendula ulmaria*)

Common names: Meadowsweet, bridewort, gravelroot, lady of the meadow, little queen, and steeple plant

Description: Queen of the meadow grows at the edges of damp woods or in roadside ditches. Its roots and rhizomes are shallow but spread lengthwise. Meadowsweet has fernlike foliage, and its leaves are dark green on the top with a white, downy undercoating. The flowers, which grow in small, irregular clusters, are off-white to white in color. The interesting thing about this plant is that the flowers and the leaves smell different from one another. The leaves have an almost vanilla-like smell, whereas the flowers smell strongly of almonds. This, in and of itself, shows that the leaves and the flowers possibly have different uses.

Parts used: Leaves and flowers

Cautions: None known

Folklore and history: Queen of the meadow has a rich history of use in the Renaissance. Culpeper wrote that it was used as a strewing herb to "make the heart glad and to delight the senses," and according to M. Grieve, meadowsweet was also one of the fifty herbs mentioned in an herbal mead, called Save, in Geoffrey Chaucer's "The Knight's Tale." Its use during the Renaissance was both magical and medicinal in nature, and it was believed that it chased away the plague and kept people healthy and wise. In some parts of England, it was thought of as a plant of impending death up until the late 1800s, and if a person were to bring a bunch of meadowsweet flowers into the house, it would mean that someone would die soon. I think this association is because during the plague meadowsweet flowers were brought in to hide the smell of death. Grieve also writes that the flowers were dried and smoked as a substitute for tobacco.

Spiritual uses: Purification, love spells, and to bring peace into a hot and stormy situation; you could strew the floor of your home with meadowsweet leaves to clean the area of negative vibrations like the people of the Renaissance period might have done. In a ritual setting, you could make an herbal tea from the leaves and asperge the circle with it or burn it on the coals to purify the area. The flowers have an association with death due to their use during the great plague, but I think the leaves are safe for love and peace because of their almond scent, which is historically associated with plants that have a love association. I have found it helpful to burn the flowers as incense during a séance, as it seems to attract the spirits of people who once loved the individuals in the room.

Spiritual anecdote: I once had a client who had an obsession with death. It was not so much that it affected her job or life, but when someone died, she was obsessed. She asked me once, "How does it feel?" and "I wonder if they were afraid?" The subject of death came up at every single session we had. On our third herbal consult, she said that there was something she hadn't told me. She told me that she felt like a worm was eating her from the inside. It sometimes caused her pain, and lately it was getting worse. We talked about things that might be causing it, and the topic of her fascination with death came up again. So, I tested a few more herbs on her, and queen of the meadow flower tested positively. Now, I usually only use queen of the meadow for people who have unresolved issues with someone who died, but I added it to her blend, and over the next few months, her fascination with death decreased. It didn't go away completely, but she was better able to deal with it. It turned out that when she was five, her dog was attacked and killed by a wolf, and she was the one to find it. She had never fully recovered from the experience.

Astrological association: Jupiter

Deities, angels, or spirit associations: Danu, Blodeuwedd, and Hecate

Meditation: Flower of darkness, open the way. Allow me to see my loved ones on the other side.

Magical spell: Take the dried flower and burn it in incense while saying the plant's meditation to help open a connection to the other worlds to talk with the dead.

Quince (*Cydonia oblonga*)

Common names: Cydonian pome, supurgillu, coyne, and apple of discord

Description: Quince is a bush-like tree that grows up to 15 feet tall and 12 feet wide. The tree has multiple trunks with deeply grooved, brownish-red bark that has knots in it. The medium green, rounded leaves grow alternating along the branches. The quince flower is white to light pink with five petals and light yellow stamens. The fruit is bright yellow and oblong in shape, being narrower at the neck than the base. The fruit has a puckered bottom.

Parts used: Fruit, seeds, and leaves

Cautions: None known

Folklore and history: In a Greek myth about quince, the goddess Eris was at a wedding and threw a quince labeled for the most beautiful in the middle of Hera, Aphrodite, and Athena, and all tried to claim it. Zeus asked Paris of Troy, the most handsome mortal man at the party, to pick the goddess the fruit belonged to, and each of the three goddesses offered him a gift. Paris picked Aphrodite's gift. This association with Aphrodite has given quince attributes of love, sexuality, and fertility. One of the traditions that was formed from this association is that a new bride had to eat a quince on the threshold of her bridal chamber, and the number of seeds in the fruit foretold how many children she would have. Another tradition, which comes from Bulgaria, is that when a baby is born, a quince tree is planted as a symbol of the cycle of life and love.

Spiritual uses: Love, happiness, fertility, and protection of relationships

Spiritual anecdote: One of the traditions I participate in is baking an apple and quince pie for bridal showers. I tell the story of Paris and Aphrodite and how the quince also protects newlyweds on their first night together. It's a magical food gift that keeps the old myths alive. I get asked to bring one to every bridal shower I'm invited to.

Astrological associations: Venus and Saturn

Deities, angels, or spirit associations: Aphrodite and Zeus

Meditation: For fertility, say: *Golden fruit of the heavens, gift me and my love many healthy children and years of love and happiness.*

Magical spell: Take a quince fruit, and while concentrating on finding true love, chant, "As I eat this fruit, my true love will come to me." Peel the fruit, cut it up, make a pie or other food with it, and eat it.

Rose (*Rosa* spp.)

Common name: Queen of Flowers

Description: The rose varies in color, but all know its design well. The flower can be red, white, or any color in between. It can have as few as five petals or as many as forty. The petals are velvety soft and exude a scent that is unmistakable. The petals fall away from the rose calyx, or rose hips, and stamens, which do not contain much scent. The flower is attached to a green stem with thorns. These thorns can face either downward or at 45-degree angles outward. Leaves also grow from these stems. They grow in groupings of three or five and have a slight rose scent. The edges of the leaves are usually a medium to dark green; the borders are lightly toothed and oblong in shape.

Parts used: Petals, rose hips, and thorns

Cautions: None known

Folklore and history: Roses are incredible plants that have been used for thousands of years to promote health, beauty, power, and mystery. It was sacred to many religions and cultures and much has been written about it in legend and myth. In Rome statues of Cupid, Venus, and Bacchus were crowned with the flowers during festivals and rites, and Romans used rose petals in everything from making wine to strewing herbs on the floor to scent the air. This flower was written about by the Greeks in countless novels and was named the "Queen of Flowers" by Sappho the Greek poetess. The rose also has quite a mystical history, and the term *sub rosa*, which means "under the rose," comes from the custom of suspending a rose over the dining table to let all know that what was said in private would go no further. It is no wonder that the rose is part of many secret societies' symbols, such as the Rosicrucianism's.

Spiritual uses: Magically, there is huge lore associated with the rose. It is, of course, seen as the flower of love, pleasure, and mirth, and the color of the flower often can determine what its magical abilities are: red for passionate love; pink for sweet, romantic love; white for innocence; and yellow for friendship. The rose has a history of being able to prevent drunkenness, which I have never tried. I have, however, taken the petals off a rose and sprinkled them on a table to do divination with—similar to how one reads tea leaves. Of course, roses can be used in any type of love-related magic, and I have used rose petals in creating a relationship incense to promote love, peace, and strength. Distilled rose water can be worn as a perfume or in your hair to attract true love, or you could place rose petals in your shoes to allow you to "walk into" the love of your life. I have used rose hips for good luck and fast-money spells, as well as in fertility magic when couples are getting tired of having intercourse by the calendar. It ignites the intensity of the act.

Spiritual anecdote: I once had a client who was a devotee of Hathor, and she was having issues with her marriage. They were mostly communication issues, but the sexual part of the relationship had disappeared for over six months. She was afraid he was with another woman and that because she was overweight and not as attractive as she used to be, she would have a hard time getting him back. Well, we started with some herbal formulas to clear up her skin and instill confidence in her because she was a beautiful woman. I had her get some rose water and told her to spray it on her sheets at night and put some in her hair during the day and before bed. I then had her burn my Lover Return to Me incense every day until her husband started acting romantic toward her. Within two weeks they were making love again, and they then went on a romantic cruise. As far as I know, their marriage is still going strong.

Astrological association: Venus

Deities, angels, or spirit associations: Aurora, Aphrodite, Astarte, Demeter, Eros, Hathor, and Isis

Meditation: Sweet smelling flower near to my heart, send me blessings for (insert wish) *so that I may be happy.*

Magical spell: Take a handful of rose petals and grind them with salt. Sprinkle the mixture in your shoes, car, purse, etc. to assist in finding true love and Mr./Ms. Right. If you just want Mr./Ms. Right Now, grind and use rose hips instead.

Rosemary (*Rosmarinus officinalis*)

Common names: Polar plant, compass weed, and compass plant

Description: Rosemary is an evergreen shrub that is native to Southern Europe. It is most often found in the dry hills of the Mediterranean. The branches have gray-colored bark that is irregular in nature, and they bear opposite, narrow, leathery, thick leaves, which are dark green above and downy white underneath. The leaves have a prominent vein in the center and edges that are rolled down. The light blue, labiate flowers grow in short axillary racemes and appear between June and July.

Parts used: Leaves, twigs, and oil

Cautions: Rosemary is a mild uterine stimulant and should be avoided during pregnancy. Excessive amounts can cause symptoms of poisoning such as nausea and vomiting.

Folklore and history: Gerard wrote that the herb "comforteth the harte and maketh it merie." It is documented that rosemary was grown in gardens as far back as the 1400s and was believed to protect the garden's owner against evil spirits. It has been used since ancient times to improve and strengthen the memory, and the Greeks would wear a sprig of it in their hair. Rosemary is also associated with fidelity, and this is one of the reasons it is often put in bridal bouquets.

Spiritual uses: Fidelity, love, healing, protection, purification, strength, virtue, and youth; it can be put under the pillow to help stop nightmares or to protect against spirits talking to you during the night. Hung over the door it keeps away thieves and harm. I mostly use it for protection, but I do make an incense for purification of my home. It contains rosemary, frankincense, white sage, and myrrh. I burn it to purify the space spiritually while I am doing physical cleaning.

Spiritual anecdote: I once had a client who had a child who had horrible night terrors. He would wake up screaming about battles and say things like his leg was cut off and he was bleeding. The mother had come to me because no one had taken her son's complaints seriously, and all they wanted to do was put him on medication. I talked to the child because I wasn't sure if it was a past life thing or a spirit talking to him. The family lived near an old cemetery with soldiers from the Civil War buried there. The child told me that he was seeing a movie behind his eyes of something that happened a long time ago. He said that it was so vivid and that a man in a dirty uniform had his leg half blown off, and he was calling out to him for help. He said he even experienced the man's pain and felt the blood on his leg. I went to the house to cleanse it and put some wards up, and I put a sprig of rosemary under his bed and told his mother to replace it weekly for at least a month. His nightmares ended within days, and last I heard, he had almost forgotten it happened. I did some education with the mother, though, because her son appears to be very sensitive to spirits. I taught her how to teach him to deal with it.

Astrological association: Sun

Deities, angels, or spirit associations: Ariadne and Belinus

Meditation: *Rosemary, sweet rosemary, give me strength and virtue, and help me to obtain my desires.*

Magical spell: Take a bundle of rosemary, tie it with a red string, and dip it in water. Use the rosemary to sprinkle water on yourself daily to stay youthful.

Rue (*Ruta graveolens*)

Common names: Garden rue, German rue, herb of grace, mother of herbs, and Ruta

Description: Rue is blue green in color and can grow up to 2 feet high. It is a summer-flowering plant, producing flowers that are small and yellow from terminal panicles. The deeply lobed leaves grow in an alternate pattern down the stem in small groupings of two or three individual lobes. There are several groupings on each stem. One of the plant's most distinguishing characteristics is its smell and taste. Rue has an acrid taste and musty smell.

Parts used: Leaves

Cautions: Can cause contact dermatitis during collection. Ingesting too much of it can cause headaches, dizziness, and gastric issues, such as nausea and vomiting. Do not ingest when pregnant or breastfeeding.

Folklore and history: Pliny tells us that rue was one of the best plants to improve sight and that people should eat it every day to keep their vision strong as they age. Victorians were fond of rue and butter finger sandwiches at tea, and it was a delicacy at many lunches. Romans trying to avert the curse of witches or the evil eye wore chaplets or crowns of rue. This plant was one that both Pagan and Catholic priests used to asperse their people with during their rites for purification and protection, especially around the time of Lammas. Historically, it was used to break hexes or curses; people would wear rue on themselves, burn it, or hang it in their homes.

Spiritual uses: Protection against curses and the evil eye, attracting money, and helping clear the mind; fresh rue, when smelled, can clear the head of lustful thinking and restore one's mind to purer thoughts. I have used it to attract fast money by burning a rue candle and carrying a leaf on me. If it grows in the garden, it is sure to protect the home against thieves and curses, as well as attract money. One of my favorite things to do with rue is to use it in warding or protecting my house. Yearly I mix rue with yarrow, ground ivy, and mullein and make herb bundles that I place around my house to protect it from curses, thieves, and lightning strikes. In small amounts it also works as a mild painkiller, especially when there is muscle damage or tension.

Spiritual anecdote: I knew a person who had pissed off a few strong magical people, and he was convinced that they had put a curse on him, so I had him make a rue candle and burn it daily to break the curse. To craft the candle, he added ground rue leaf to the wax as well as some rue essential oil right before he poured it into the melting pot and chanted some simple protective charms. He added green coloring and poured it into a jar. He then painted a protective symbol on the candle and burned it every day until the candle was gone. Within a few days of burning it, his luck returned to normal. You can buy rue candles at magical stores, but nothing beats making your own, putting the intention into it, and then using it.

Astrological association: Mars

Deities, angels, or spirit associations: Aradia, Diana, and Pan

Meditation: *O herb of grace, help protect me against my enemies and keep me safe from harm.*

Magical spell: Take a sprig of rue, yarrow, mullein, and ground ivy, tie them together at one end, and hang the bundle in a window of your home. Do this for each window in your home. Make another bundle and hang it either above the front door or under the threshold. These bundles will protect your home from curses, the evil eye, thieves, and lightning.

Sage (*Salvia officinalis*)

Common names: Broadleaf sage, garden sage, and sawge

Description: Sage is a perennial, herbaceous to shrubby herb that grows up to 20 inches in height. It is native to the Balkans and the Mediterranean but is grown widely elsewhere as a garden and pot herb. Sage has a woody stem and lower branches. These branches give way to the square stem, which is green or purplish and covered in a fine down. The stalked and opposite leaves are oblong to lanceolate, have a leathery texture, and are covered in fine down. The leaf is gray and has delicately toothed margins. The blueish-purple flowers, which appear in June and July, have two lips and a white throat. The flowers develop at the end of a spike at the tip of the stem and grow in a whorl pattern around the stem.

Parts used: Leaves and essential oil

Cautions: According to Blumenthal in *The Complete German Commission E Monographs*, alcoholic extracts of sage have a high concentration of thujone, which can be toxic in large doses. Avoid ingesting sage during pregnancy because it is a uterine stimulant. Small doses of the essential oil can be poisonous when ingested.

Folklore and history: This herb's name comes from the Latin *salvere*, meaning "to save," which is in reference to its healing powers. In the Middle Ages in England, a common saying was "he that would live for aye, must eat sage in May," and it was also said that this plant would thrive or wither just as its owner's business would prosper or fail. An old French saying is "Sage helps the nerves and by its powerful might palsy is cured and fever put to flight." Gerard said it was good for the bite and sting of sea serpents, and John Baptista Porta wrote that garden sage mixed with gemstones and gold would cause immortality.

Spiritual uses: Healing, immortality, protection against the evil eye, and wisdom

Spiritual anecdote: Sage is a subtle protector that seems to keep a low profile until it's needed most. I had a student who was getting divorced, and her husband was being petty, but then it came to the custody of their children, which is when things got ugly. He tried to take her children away from her, claiming that she wasn't a good mother because she was a Pagan. It was right before Thanksgiving, and she was talking to her herbs, including her sage, and she asked them to give her wisdom on what to do to protect her in this circumstance. Now, a few things happened all at once. Her sage plant—within a few days—doubled its size, and her husband choked on a sage leaf stem in some stuffing at Thanksgiving. For some reason, he was less willing to take away the children after this. Sage does not mess around when it is called upon to protect you.

Astrological association: Jupiter

Deities, angels, or spirit associations: Apollo, Belinus, Athena, and Brigantia

Meditation: *Herb of wisdom, herb of protection, keep me from the negativity of my enemies.*

Magical spells: Keep a sage leaf on you at all times for protection against the evil eye and to help promote wisdom. Make a tea with one leaf daily to promote a long life.

Saint John's Wort (*Hypericum perforatum*)

Common names: Amber, *Fuga daemonum*, goat weed, herba John, John's wort, Saint John's girdle, and tipton weed

Description: Saint John's wort reaches up to 2 feet tall, growing in pastures, at forest edges, and along roadsides. It has bright yellow flowers that start blooming on or around Saint John's day, June 24, and last until August. The flowers have five petals with multiple stamens in the center and grow in small bunches. The leaves are small, light green, and oblong. When held up to the light, both the leaves and the flowers have what appear to be holes, which are actually visible oil glands. The flowers produce small black seeds, which are held in a multiple-celled container. The plant can be an invasive weed in disturbed ground and is considered toxic to grazing cattle.

Parts used: Flowers and upper leaves

Cautions: Do not ingest if you are on any type of medicine, especially blood pressure, antibiotics, antidepressants, transplant, or hormonal birth control medicines.

Folklore and history: Saint John's wort has quite a history when it comes to repelling Witchcraft or evil magic. Its Latin name means "over an apparition," which means that it was a strong repellent to evil spirits and that just the smell of it would cause them to run. I find it funny that during the Renaissance the church used this herb to determine who was or wasn't a witch, as I think that most of the herbs that were supposed to protect against witches were actually protectors of the witches and herbalists. A common story that is told about Saint John's wort, which is actually how it got its name, is that Saint John was walking through the forest and was surrounded by wild beasts and evil spirits. To protect himself, he made a girdle of the plant.

Spiritual uses: As an herb that protects witches and herbalists, Saint John's wort is a great ally to have. I have this herb hanging in my house to protect me against people that may try to cause me harm, as well as to protect my house against lightning strikes, which is one of its older magical uses. I make a witch bottle with Saint John's wort, yarrow, and mullein, along with brightly colored glass pebbles, and give it to new homeowners to protect their home against thieves, lightning strikes, and harmful spirits. Saint John's wort is also a favorite herb of the fey, and if you plant it in your garden, you are sure to attract them and keep them around. I've planted at least one bush every place I have ever lived to attract nature spirits and keep the peace with the fey.

This herb has another major magical attribute, and it relates to the holes or pores in the leaves and flowers. To me, this signature relates to the herb's ability to release obstacles and open doorways either in this world or the next. It can be burned in incense during astral travel or journey work to help you reach that next level. I make an oil from the flowers, which turns red when infused in the sun; this oil can be used as a blood substitute. I apply the oil when I am planning on doing some astral travel or journey work to help open doors to other worlds.

Spiritual anecdote: I have a friend who constantly lost things, and she kept on blaming it on "evil spirits." So, I made her a magical bag, and one of the main ingredients was Saint John's wort. I told her to make sure she had a fir tree on her property or other conifer tree for the fey to live in during the winter. I also told her to leave jelly beans out when she needs to find something. I think her issue was that the fey were torturing her because she disliked nature had paved most of her property, and the spirits of land were not happy with her. The Saint John's wort and the jelly beans were to help satisfy some of these mischievous spirits.

Astrological association: Sun

Deities, angels, or spirit associations: Baldur, Saint John, the fey, and Thor

Meditation: Herb of protection, protect me against people who would harm me and keep me safe.

Magical spell: Take the oil of Saint John's wort and apply it to your temples, carotids, and wrists before astral traveling. The oil will ease your way into other states as well as protect you on your journey.

Sandalwood (*Santalum album*)

Common names: Yellow sandalwood and Indian sandalwood

Description: The sandalwood tree grows up to 30 feet tall. It is a hemiparasitic tree, meaning it relies on nutrients from other trees and grasses around it to survive, and its roots wrap themselves around other trees' roots to extract nutrients from them. The bark on the outer layer is dark brown, but underneath the outer bark is yellow-brown heartwood. The dark green leaves are slightly shiny and grow equally up the stems. The flowers grow at the end of each stem in a panicle pattern. They are four petaled and initially are light green in color but then turn red. The berries are dark red and have small light brown seeds. The trees are usually harvested between fifteen and twenty years of age, and all wood parts of the tree are used, including the roots.

Parts used: Wood, including roots

Cautions: None known

Folklore and history: Sandalwood has been used for spiritual purposes since before there was written language in India, and it is written about in the Vedas, which is one of India's oldest and most sacred texts. It has been burned in incense for thousands of years in India, Egypt, and the Middle East. One of my favorite myths is how Ganesh was created. His mother, the goddess Parvati, wanted a child, so she took some of the sandalwood paste that she used for her bath, mixed it with clay, and breathed life into it. In the Hindu religion, sandalwood is ground into a powder and water is added to make a paste. This paste sometimes has saffron added to give it a red color. After some ceremonies or rituals, the paste is put over the third eye region to help one connect with the Divine or to calm the mind. In Buddhism sandalwood incense is often offered during worship and is associated with keeping focused during meditation. There are some religions that have associated the tree as a funerary one and either burn the incense as part of funeral rites or apply the oil to the body; it is thought to help the spirit transition to the other side. Many of the large sacred statues of deities and Buddha at temples are carved from sandalwood. One of the largest that I have seen in person was a Buddha statue 30 feet tall and at least 10 feet wide at the base, gilded with gold and colorful paints.

Spiritual uses: Connecting to the Divine, spiritual focus, calmness, transitions, trance work, divination, and purification; I love the scent of sandalwood, and I use it whenever I am feeling not as connected to the Divine as I like would like or when I am stressed and not able to get to a good place mentally. I also burn sandalwood incense when I do trance work. There are the spiritual and calming effects of burning it, and according to modern science, there is also a biochemical reaction in our primal brain when one of these sacred scents is used.

Spiritual anecdote: One of my clients owns a yoga studio, and one day she talked about how she has a swami come to her studio once a month to teach meditation. He burns incense as an offering to Ganesh before every session, saying that honoring him in this way connects with him and removes obstacles that often happen when people try to meditate. The scent of sandalwood incense made my client easily slip into the meditative state she needed to be in and helped her connect to the Divine.

Astrological association: Jupiter

Deities, angels, or spirit associations: Parvati, Shiva, and Ganesh

Meditation: *Sacred tree, purify and guide me as I journey to other worlds to hear the universe's wisdom.*

Magical spell: Before trance work, burn sandalwood incense and mix some sandalwood powder in enough rose water or hydrosol to make a thick paste. Dab some on your third eye and at the top of your head on your crown chakra. Inhale a breath lasting three seconds, hold it for two seconds, and exhale to a count of three seconds. Repeat this eight times. After this breathing meditation, begin the trance work or astral travel that you plan on doing.

Solomon's Seal (*Polygonatum multiflorum*)

Common names: Lady's seal and Saint Mary's seal

Description: Solomon's seal can grow to be more than 36 inches tall and is indistinct until it flowers around midsummer, as the distinctive feature in identifying this plant is the placement of the flowers and its berries. The leaves are lanced shaped and dark green. They grow in an alternate pattern. The flowers are white to cream in color and grow underneath the leaf axial on the central stem. The flowers remind me of tiny fairy bells, and they produce big, juicy, bluish-black berries with multiple seeds in them. The rhizomes, which are the parts that are used medicinally, are white and fleshy. In fact, the rhizomes look like finger bones with knuckles or vertebrae. The best time to harvest this plant is in the early fall, after the berries have fallen off and the leaves start to turn brown.

Parts used: Roots and rhizomes

Cautions: None known

Folklore and history: Spiritually there isn't much written about this herb, and I mostly learned about its spiritual side from talking to my Dakota teachers and by using it. I was taught that it can help one escape harm from demons by making you invisible to them. In order to do this, the root needs to be harvested in July with a tobacco offering, dried, and then stored in red flannel wrapped with a blue thread. The root can only be used once for protection, and after it is used, it needs to be buried in the flannel under an oak tree with some tobacco and prayed over. If this funeral ritual is not done, I was told that the protection the root provides will never work again.

Spiritual uses: Protection, exorcisms, shape-shifting, and increasing wealth; Solomon's seal is an excellent herb to burn in incense blends for exorcism of spirits, bad habits, or negative energies. I have also used it in money magic, as the root can be sliced and carried in your wallet or pocket to increase wealth.

Spiritual anecdote: I have used Solomon's seal a lot for arthritis in my herbal practice, and one day I met this child who was eight years old with cramped-up fingers that looked like rheumatism, but it wasn't. The mother had taken the child in for all kinds of testing, and nothing came out positive. So, I spoke to the child's parent some more and found out that her child liked to steal things, especially from friends, as well as pull hair. This behavior, of course, had led to hours of counseling, and the child kept saying that he couldn't help it—something just came over him when they saw brightly colored objects or toys he wanted, and he liked to pull hair. At first I was thinking maybe this was a fey possession, but I tried fey-repelling herbs, and they didn't test well. So, I was thinking that since his fingers resembled that of Solomon's seal root, and sometimes herbs that look like a body part work on that body part, I would try it. The herb worked, getting him to stop pulling hair, and it healed his fingers. A year or so later, I asked my Dakota teacher about it, and she said that Solomon's seal is used for children who are possessed by a not-so-nice Great Plains spirit that likes to steal and pull hair. She had a name for it, but she translated it into "the grabby spirit."

Astrological association: Moon

Deities, angels, or spirit associations: White Buffalo Calf Woman and thunder spirits

Meditation: Root of Solomon, help me obtain the money I need to live like King Solomon.

Magical spell: For shape-shifting, drink a tisane of the root an hour or so before you want to change form. For this, I usually mix it with kava and cinnamon.

Sweetgrass (*Hierochloe odorata*)

Common names: Holy grass, hair of the mother, manna grass, and vanilla grass

Description: Sweetgrass is a slender grass that grows in a clumping pattern and spreads by rhizomes. The flat, bright green leaves grow up to 2 feet long and grow directly from the ground. The leaves are shiny underneath and matte on the top. The grass flowers in the late summer from multiple stems that come from the ground. On these stems, multiple small cream-colored flowers with three to four small petals form. The seeds are very small and light brown.

Parts used: Leaves

Cautions: None known

Folklore and history: Sweetgrass is one of the four sacred herbs of many Native American tribes, the other herbs being tobacco, white sage, and cedar. Sweetgrass is known as the "hair of the mother" because its sweet scent wraps people in its love like a mother would. Sweetgrass is traditionally used as a cleansing plant after white sage or cedar have been used, as it brings good energies back into a space after white sage or cedar rids it of negative energies.

Spiritual uses: Bringing good energy to a space after purification, adding sweetness to life, and loving yourself; I like to add this to purification spells or to spells that aim to bring happiness to people, especially after a loss.

Spiritual anecdote: I had a client who could only pay with tobacco, fresh sweetgrass, and other plants. She would come see me every six months or so, and I would always welcome her late summer visits because she would bring me fresh sweetgrass, which I would braid and give as gifts during the holidays. One day I asked her if she ever used the sweetgrass that she harvested for herself, and she said that she did not. My client had lost her husband about three years before I started seeing her, and she still went to her shaman's sweat lodge, as it helped her deal with the grief for a while. Around the holidays, my client came to the herb store to buy supplies, and I happened to have one of the sweetgrass braids on hand. I gifted it to her and told her that she needed to bring sweetness into her life. She started crying and told me that one of the things she missed about her husband the most was that he used to braid her hair and sometimes weave a few blades of sweetgrass into it. I reminded her that it would help her if she cleansed with smoke on every full moon and added that she should burn some of the sweetgrass I had braided with love to help her bring some sweetness into her life.

Astrological association: Mercury

Deities, angels, or spirit associations: Earth spirits and White Buffalo Calf Woman

Meditation: As you burn sweetgrass, say: *Mother, take my burning of this sweetgrass as proof of my love of you and your children and help me bring more sweetness in my life.*

Magical spell: Mix equal parts dried rose petals, sweetgrass, and sandalwood together and burn on a charcoal to help with recovery from addiction.

Sweet Gum (*Liquidamber styraciflua*)

Common names: Witches' balls, liquid amber, red gum tree, alligator tree, and American storax

Description: The sweet gum tree grows 80 to 100 feet tall; it grows very straight and has a grayish-brown bark that has deep vertical grooves in it. Sweet gum likes to grow in damp areas and has a shallow but wide root system. The leaves are medium green, glossy, and palmate or star shaped with lightly toothed margins. They turn a beautiful red/orange in the fall and will drop in the winter. The flowers are small and yellow and grow up in a panicle or cone at the end of the branch. Each one of the flowers matures into the most interesting part of this tree, which is the spiky seedpods. The seedpods are brown and have many spiny protrusions. If you were to open one, you would see small dark brown seeds with small winglike protrusions that allow them to fly on the winds to create more trees.

Parts used: Seedpods, resin, and leaves

Cautions: Do not eat the sweet gum ball; it is a choking hazard.

Folklore and history: These trees have a history of being used to make storax, a common gumlike resin that is used in manufacturing as a thickening agent. Traditionally, the sap was tapped, like how maple trees are tapped to make syrup, and the same process is used today. The wood is very strong and reddish, so woodworkers often used it to make furniture. The balls were gathered in the fall and placed under stairs and in the way of people who would wish to harm the user.

Spiritual uses: When it comes to sweet gum, it's the seedpods that are traditionally used for magic. You can protect yourself with them by putting the spiky balls around your home or carrying them with you. In hoodoo these balls are put in bags to be carried for protection or put into jars, and you could make a witch bottle with the seedpods, rusty nails, and urine to protect yourself against negative spirits. Just remember that witch bottles do need to be buried in the corner of your property because they will crack or explode over time. Care should always be taken when working with urine and any other bodily fluids too. The seedpods are much more useful for keeping away spirits and demons than protecting against a person—unless that person is possessed or acting on some negative spirit's behalf. The seedpods also have the ability to keep away mischievous spirits/fey that want to come into the house, and I have used the balls to create ornamental and protective garlands for the front door for this purpose. The leaves of the sweet gum tree can be dried and used for incense. They have a sweet, resinous smell.

Spiritual anecdote: I know an older native Floridian who places sweet gum trees along the edge of her property for protection. She gathers the balls and puts them under her stairs to keep any mischievous teenagers from coming to knock on her front door.

Astrological association: Uranus

Deities, angels, or spirit associations: Amaterasu and Hachiman

Meditation: *Tree so tall and strong, protect me as I walk my path and keep me from harm.*

Magical spell: For protection, take a small jar and put a sweet gum ball in it. Add a rusty nail, a razor, if you have one, and some rose thorns, if you have them. Fill the jar ⅔ of the way up with urine, being careful when working with the fluid, and seal the jar. Go to a far corner of your property and bury the bottle at least 1 foot deep. This jar will protect you against people and spirits that want to harm you.

Tea (*Camellia sinensis*)

Common names: Green tea, black tea, oolong tea, *Thea sinensis*, and jassamica

Description: This small evergreen shrub is grown in Sri Lanka, Java, Japan, and other regions where the climate allows. It grows to a height of 6 feet when cultivated but may reach 20 feet high in the wild. The dark green lanceolate leaves grow on short stalks. They are blunt at the apex with a tapering base and mildly serrate margins. The young leaves are hairy, while the older ones are glabrous. The white flowers, which have multiple yellow stamens, droop from short stalks. They can be solitary, or several can occur together on short branchlets in between the leaf axils. The fruit is a smooth, flat, round, and three-celled capsule with a single seed in each cell.

Parts used: Dried and rolled leaf buds and very young leaves

Cautions: Excessive quantities may cause nervous symptoms including agitation, palpitations, and irritability. Pregnant and nursing women should limit their consumption to two cups a day.

Folklore and history: Tea has a long history of use in Asia, and it was brought to Europe via the spice road and has been a staple beverage ever since. Different types of tea are actually from the same plant. They are just processed differently. The green tea leaves are allowed to wither in hot air before they're sautéed in a pan to stop the fermentation processes. The leaves of oolong are wilted in sunlight, lightly bruised, and allowed to partially darken until reddening of the leaf edges occurs. Black tea leaves are fermented in cool, humid rooms until the leaf is oxidized. White tea is the least processed; it is just allowed to air-dry and not ferment. The myth of how tea came to be began in China more than five thousand years ago. According to legend, the mythological emperor Shen Nung required that all drinking water be boiled as a precaution against disease. One summer, he stopped to rest near a large bush. His servants began to boil water and a few leaves from the bush fell into the boiling water. The emperor was curious about this new liquid, drank some, and found it very refreshing. And so, according to this legend, tea was invented.

Spiritual uses: Tea has the ability to create great strength and courage in the person who drinks it. It can burned in incense or consumed as a tea in aphrodisiac magic. I have made an aphrodisiac tea with black tea, rose petals, and jasmine flowers to drink and give to my love to promote endurance and romance. If a tea leaf is carried, it will help promote wealth, and it will keep the person carrying it courageous. I have also burned it as incense to promote courage in someone who was about to go into a job interview.

Spiritual anecdote: When I worked at an herb store, I had the pleasure of being able to mix herbs with tea to produce certain results for the customers. One of these customers wanted a special tea to serve to party guests that would help them feel like they were giddy with happiness because she said they were too serious to have any fun with. For this request, I mixed a tea and herb blend that had green tea, damiana, blue corn flowers, and lemon balm. She served the tea, and she said that everyone liked the tea blend and that her guests were laughing and enjoying themselves.

Astrological association: Sun

Deities, angels, or spirit associations: Quan Yin and Lugh

Meditation: Sweet herb, sweet love, open the doors to pleasure and help my desires and the desires of my love grow.

Magical spells: Drink it as a tea for its aphrodisiac and courage-promoting properties or carry it for wealth, courage, or love. Mix black tea, red rose petals, and jasmine flowers together for an aphrodisiac drink that will improve performance, endurance, and closeness.

Thorn Apple (*Datura stramonium*)

Common names: Datura, Devil's-apple, Jamestown weed, Jimsonweed, stinkweed, Devil's trumpet, and apple of Peru

Description: Thorn apple is a beautiful plant that can grow up to 5 feet tall and 4 feet wide. The stem is thick and green with streaks of purple throughout. The leaves are 3 to 5 inches long and ovate with irregular protruding lobes that have a fetid smell. The large trumpet-shaped flower blooms at night, is up to 3½ inches long, is white to light purple in color, and grows facing upward. One of the most distinguishing features of the plant is its seedpod. It is round to egg shaped and covered with sharp thorns. When the pod splits open, it resembles a four-petaled flower. The seedpod, when ripe, contains up to one hundred brown to black seeds.

Parts used: Leaves, flowers, and seeds

Cautions: Do not eat or drink due to its toxicity; wash your hands after handling it in case you rub your eyes or accidentally ingest it.

Folklore and history: Even in the time of Dioscorides, thorn apple was known as a powerful plant that in small doses could cure disease and in larger amounts led to hallucinations and/or death. He states that "the root being drunk with wine in the quantity of a dram has the power to effect unpleasant fantasies. But two being drunk, make one beside himself for three days and four being drunk kill him." *Datura* comes from the Sanskrit word *dhattura*, which was a word for members of an ancient religious sect that worshipped Kali. They used a species of datura native to India to drug the soon-to-be-sacrificed victims to the dark goddess. It is theorized that the priestesses at the Oracle of Delphi might have used the leaves as part of their incense blend. When the American settlers arrived at Jamestown, a few of the men went out and ate some of this plant and came back to the village stark raving mad, hence one of its common names—Jamestown weed. The flowers of this plant are its most toxic. They can be up to 0.61 percent of the alkaloid hyoscyamine. The seeds, which are the second most toxic part, can have up to 0.58 percent of the poison. This plant can be quite deadly, and it is not recommended for use. Overdose can be obtained by ingesting as little as one hundred seeds or 1 gram of datura flower.

Spiritual uses: Thorn apple is an interesting magical and medicinal plant that has a greater use in history than in modern times due to its toxic effects. Traditionally, it was used as an ingredient in flying ointment, but even in small doses it is dangerous. Even smelling the flower is enough to cause a mild intoxication; I use the flowers during dark moon rituals or on Samhain as an altar decoration.

Spiritual anecdote: I use this plant very carefully because it is poisonous, but I feel that, as an herbalist, I should know or have experience with all of the plants around me because they also have medicinal properties. I do use the flowers to make flying ointment, and I am careful about how much of the plant I use in the formula.

Astrological association: Mars

Deities, angels, or spirit associations: Kali and Lucifer

Meditation: Sister of the darkness, open up and let me in to see the other side of the light, let me see the truth within.

Magical spell: Take a leaf, wrap it up with red thread, and put it in a plastic baggie. Carry it with you when you plan to astral travel. It will help get you there.

Tobacco (*Nicotina tabacum*)

Common names: Tobacca and tobacco folia

Description: Tobacco is an annual herb that reaches 4 to 6 feet tall. Its leaves are a medium green on top and pale green on the underside. Tobacco's leaves grow quite large, sometimes getting up to 2 feet long, and are ovate in nature. Tobacco flowers during the summer. Its flowers are red to rose-colored and grow off panicles at the end of the stems.

Parts used: Cured and dried leaves

Cautions: Do not ingest; it can cause nausea and dizziness. Do not use in excess.

Folklore and history: Native Americans have used tobacco as a sacred plant for hundreds of years. It was smoked to seal deals, at powwows among the elders as an act of peace, and at ceremonies as an offering to the gods. It was first exported to England in 1586, where it became popular as a snuff and then as an herb to smoke. Initially it was unpopular. Kings prohibited it, the pope rallied against it, and, in the East, sultans killed those who smoked it. By the 1800s tobacco was all the rage across Europe and widely smoked.

Spiritual uses: Tobacco has several magical applications, but I personally only use one or two because the plant itself has a very old and powerful spirit. This sacred herb should not be used lightly, without permission of the tobacco plant spirit, or in excess once that permission has been obtained. The most common thing I use tobacco for is an offering to other plant spirits when I am wildcrafting. I usually talk to the plant before I harvest it and ask it what it would like for an offering. One of the things some plant spirits ask for is tobacco. I have also used it as an offering to certain gods I have asked requests of. This usually works best for African deities and some of the more ancient god/goddess forms. It can be burned in incense to create a powerful purification aid, which will get rid of all negativities and all spirits—good and bad. If using tobacco for this purpose, follow it with sweetgrass, which will bring in the good and protective spirits. It can also be smoked as an offering to certain gods and can help you communicate with them. Use tobacco in moderation and with great respect to its plant spirit. Overuse can cause serious illness and death.

Spiritual anecdote: I have a variety of gods and spirits that call to me. One of them is an African deity, and when he is near, I need to smoke a cigar and drink some rum. Now, once I was dealing with a woman who was a little dishonest, and she evidently had angered some powerful Santerían people and was having a lot of magic work being done against her. Well, we were in a business deal together, and I kept having this deity come to me, telling me to go smoke outside. What I saw through the exhaled smoke was a beast of some sort at the edge of my property with red eyes. It could not get to me because my land is heavily warded, but the spirit showed me that if I got into a serious business deal with her, her fate would be mine. I ended the relationship a short time after seeing that vision to avoid any issues.

Astrological association: Mars

Deities, angels, or spirit associations: Baron Samedi, elementals, plant spirits, and many African deities

Meditation: Powerful one, grant me your protection and shield me from harm; protect me from my enemies both seen and unseen.

Magical spell: Take a tobacco leaf and wrap it with red thread while chanting the plant's meditation. Carry it with you for general protection against harmful people and spirits.

Valerian (*Valeriana officinalis*)

Common names: Allheal, amantilla, capon's taile, cat's valerian, English valerian, and *phu*

Description: Valerian grows between 2 and 3 feet tall. The leaves are medium green and grow bilaterally along the green stem in six to ten pairs per stem. The leaves reach 3 to 4 inches long with saw-toothed borders and have a mild odor. I think the flowers on this plant are absolutely beautiful. They are small and white with a pink tinge to them and grow in a cluster at the top of each plant. The flowers have the characteristic smell of valerian root, only milder and sweeter. The root grows to be 1 to 2 feet long and sends out horizontal rhizomes, which grow into more plants. The root is dark brown and is nondescript except for its smell, which some people have likened to sweaty socks.

Parts used: Roots

Cautions: Use with caution if using with alcohol or relaxants of any kind as it can strengthen any narcotics.

Folklore and history: This plant was used as far back as Dioscorides for both medicine and magic. One of my favorite comments comes from Pliny, who says it's good for the bite of any venomous creature, including sea serpents. It was often known as the "witch's herbe" as it banished all evil influences including the plague. Most of its lore is around protection and love magic; it is said that if you wear it, all men will flock to you to do your bidding.

Spiritual uses: Cat magic, protection, and chasing demons away; this herb can be used with cat familiars as well as spirit guides of the feline persuasion. It can be given as an offering to Bast or any other feline entity prior to magical work or after a job has been completed as a reward. If you choose to use valerian in magic, I recommend that you do not burn it in incense because its smell is intensely unpleasant. However, if you were trying to chase a negative spirit or demon from the house, this would do the trick. I have heard of people burning it in haunted houses, where nothing else worked, with excellent results. I use it for dream workings and love magic.

Spiritual anecdote: I have a friend who is a devotee of Bast, and she was having a run of bad luck. She told me that she had been putting out catnip as an offering, but nothing was happening. She also told me that she was having trouble sleeping because her mind kept racing. I suggested she leave out a plate with valerian root on it instead and take a valerian flower from my garden to put on Bast's altar. I also told her to make herself an herbal tea with valerian, peppermint, and California poppy to drink before bed. The next week she called me saying that her luck was changing for the better and that she was able to get to sleep with no problems.

Astrological association: Mercury

Deities, angels, or spirit associations: Bast, Sekhmet, and Aphrodite

Meditation: Root so deep and dark, bring to light the love of my life and show them the way to me so that we both may be happy.

Magical spell: For love magic, take a piece of the root and bind it with pink thread while chanting the plant's incantation to attract true love to you. Take that root and carry it with you in a pink or red pouch.

Vervain (*Verbena officinalis*)

Common names: Verbena, britannica, enchanter's plant, herb of enchantment, herb of grace, holy herb, *herba sacra*, Juno's tears, simpler's-joy, and pigeon wood

Description: Vervain is a tall, noble-looking plant with square stems and alternate leaves. It grows to be 2½ to 3 feet tall and is easily identified by its tall, purple-blue spires, which rise above the grasses. These pencil-shaped flower spikes, which can grow up to 8 inches in length, are the plant's most distinguishing feature. The blue-violet flowers of the vervain plant are small and four petaled. The leaves are medium green in color and grow unequally along the stem. The leaves are 1 to 2 inches in length and have even and regular saw-toothed edges. Both blue vervain and vervain can be used interchangeably for magical acts.

Parts used: Leaves, flowers, and stems

Cautions: None known

Folklore and history: In 1523 Gerard wrote that it was recommended that people drink iron water and vervain to dry up worms, open up a stopped liver, and calm fears. Galen said that vervain should be gathered in the hour of Venus when her moon is in Libra for optimum strength and that whoever carries vervain in their hands will not be barked at by dogs. The oracle at the Temple of Apollo in Delphi supposedly used vervain in one of the incense blends to train new oracles, as well as to help induce a trance in the Pythia. Priests in Rome used an infusion of vervain to clean the altars of Jupiter on Thursdays. Legend says that in order to remain chaste for seven years, wake up and gather vervain before the sun rises on the solstice, press the juice out of the stems, and drink it. According to the legend, the juice will cause you to lose sexual desire for seven full years. The juice of the vervain plant smeared on the body is said to fulfill every wish, help you see into the future, turn enemies into friends, attract lovers, and protect you against all enchantments. A salve made of the juice of vervain, hog's lard, and other herbs was used to induce a trance in European shamanic traditions. An old folk tradition to make iron stronger was to put vervain in the water that the smiths quenched the iron in, and that tradition is still used by some craftspeople today to increase the magical strength of their tools.

Spiritual uses: Love, protection, truth, peace, money, purification, and healing; a crown of vervain will protect against danger while invoking spirits, as well as calm extreme emotions. An infusion sprinkled around the house will chase off negative forces and spirits. If someone you know has taken something from you, wear vervain when you confront the person and they will be unable to lie to you. Vervain can also be used as a protective device for your home. For this purpose, I suggest that the herb be used in a dried flower arrangement above the front door or burned in incense to protect against negative spirits or persons entering the home. I have also added a few dried vervain heads to my magical broom to assist in sweeping out harmful influences prior to ritual. Vervain loses some of its medicinal qualities when dried, but this does not affect its magical properties.

Spiritual anecdote: One of the magical gifts I make for new high priestesses is a crown of vervain. It enhances the trancelike state and encourages communication with deities. I also give each new priestess a bottle of vervain tincture to take prior to drawing down the goddess. This tincture relaxes them and opens all their chakras, especially their third eye. One of these priestesses, whom I gifted with a crown, later told me that she normally had a hard time drawing down, but the first time she wore it, she easily fell into the trancelike state needed and had an excellent experience.

Astrological association: Venus

Deities, angels, or spirit associations: Gabriel, Apollo, Aphrodite, Aradia, Zeus, Thor, Hera, and Cerridwen

Meditation: Herb of Venus, herb of grace, grant me the skill to see the future, give me the wisdom to know what to do with the knowledge, and give me the strength to speak the visions you bring me.

Magical spells: Before ritual, brew a vervain tisane using a teaspoon of vervain in a cup of water. Steep it for twenty minutes, sweeten as needed, and then say the plant's meditation while concentrating on connecting with the gods or the universal energies. I also use a cup of this tisane to bathe my magical tools and altar with to clean them spiritually. If you add mugwort to the mix, it can be used with scrying tools to clean them and help them give clearer visions.

Vetiver (*Chrysopogon zizanioides*)

Common names: Khus and wonder grass

Description: Vetiver grass has a very deep root system that forms in a clump of rootlets, called a crown, that can grow up to 9 feet deep and 3 feet wide. The roots are light brown and thin with multiple branches that weave through each other. The leaves, which grow in clumps from the underground crown, can reach 5 feet tall. They are medium green, rounded at the base, and flat at the top. The leaves are strong and ridged. They stand straight up until the top of the leaf, which starts to bend. The flower stems grow directly from the ground, and at the tops of these stems, the plant produces whorls of small hairy branches, which produce very small brownish-purple flowers that have three petals and open only slightly. An interesting fact about this grass is that it can live to be one hundred years old and can grow nearly anywhere, including salty marshes. This property, plus the strength of the plant's leaves, shows us what it can be used for.

Parts used: Roots and essential oil

Cautions: None known

Folklore and history: Vetiver is the Tamil word for "root that is dug up," and it has been used in the perfume industry for centuries. In fact, as far back as the twelfth century, vetiver was used in the Indian perfume industry and was referred to as the "oil of tranquility." While the roots are used in

India's perfume industry, the leaves have one-sixth the tensile strength of steel and are used to thatch roofs and make ropes. The grass is often woven into garlands, which are used as an offering to Shiva and Ganesh during Hindu festivals, while the incense made of the root powder is burned as an offering.

Spiritual uses: Strength, longevity, growth, fertility, promoting calmness, and reducing stress

Spiritual anecdote: I used to work with a woman whose mother was a traditional Haitian healer. She used to grow the plant, harvest the roots, and add them to oil to make an infusion that could be used for everything from cooling a fever to bringing money into your life. I was lucky enough to get a small jar of this magical oil, and it was amazing. I had a client who had PTSD, and it was severe to the extent that if a door slammed, he would jump from fear. In addition to using some herbs and teaching him to meditate, I gave him a small vial of this oil to carry with him. He would take a drop of it and rub it into his hair whenever he thought he would be in a situation that would trigger his PTSD. He said that it seemed to help him, and because I couldn't grow this magical grass in Minnesota, I had him buy the essential oil of vetiver grass to carry with him. He added that the oil also helped him stop snoring, which made his wife happy.

Astrological association: Saturn

Deities, angels, or spirit associations: Ganesh and Shiva

Meditation: Grass with roots so deep, give me the strength to get through these trying times and help lift me to a better place.

Magical spells: Use the essential oil to anoint a candle dedicated to Ganesh, who will help you remove obstacles. Take the oil and wear it during meditation to help calm the mind and remain focused on the meditation.

Violet (*Viola odorata*)

Common name: Sweet violet

Description: Violets rarely reach more than 1 foot tall and grow in part shade, often appearing in forest clearings, damp meadows, or pastures. They usually grow in colonies, and the parts that are usually harvested are the leaves and flowers. The leaves are heart shaped, dark green, and covered with soft, fine hairs. The violet flower is deep purple and interesting in that it has five unequal petals and five sepals, which combine into a narrow tube at the base. Another interesting feature about the flower is that the beautiful purple flowers you see in the spring serve no reproductive use. The violet plant bears a second set of flowers in the early fall that are small and inconspicuous and have no petals. These flowers are the ones that produce seeds. Those seeds aren't the only way the violet plant reproduces; it also reproduces by sending underground runners.

Parts used: Leaves and flowers

Cautions: None known

Folklore and history: The violet has some interesting mythology and history behind it. In one Greek myth, Zeus has a romantic affair with a water nymph, Io, and when Hera finds out about it, she threatens to kill her. Because of Hera's anger, Zeus turns Io into a white heifer in order to hide her. Io doesn't like the tough grass she has to eat, though, so Zeus, feeling sorry for her, turns her tears into violets, which she is then able to eat instead of grass.

Another story related to the flower goes back to Napoleon. It seems that when Napoleon went to Elba, his followers adopted the violet as their secret symbol because he promised that he would "return in the spring with the violets." He kept his promise and returned to Paris that following May. Violets were also mentioned by both Virgil and Homer as remedies for anger and to strengthen the heart.

Spiritual uses: Magically, violets are wonderful to add to your palette of herbs. One of the things that violets are capable of doing is bringing back simple joy and peace. To incorporate this herb into a magical act, drink it in a tea blend or burn it in incense for ritual. Other things that violets are used for are fertility or to find out the gender of your child. You can drink a tea for this or put a violet leaf under your pillow, and the gender you dream about when you sleep will be the gender of the child. Violet leaves and flowers can also be used in love magic. For this you can drink it in a tea or make syrup with it and give it to the person you desire in hopes that they will express their love for you.

I make a flower syrup when the flowers are in bloom to capture their essence, so I have it when I need it. I use it for love, healing, peace, happiness, and protection magic. My favorite thing to use it for is in fairy magic because they are very attracted to the violet flower syrup. I take a shot glass, fill it with the violet syrup, and put it on my altar, and it is usually gone the next day. I often find a gift nearby.

Spiritual anecdote: I once had an herbal client who had breast cancer. She was going through chemotherapy and came to me to help boost her immune system. She also could not be happy about anything, and she was wondering if there was any herb that could be used to restore her happiness. I tested a few herbs on her, and violet flower tested really well. I added it to her formula because it also helps with the lymphatic system. Then, I asked her if she had a patch of violets that she could go to and sit in and just be with the flowers. She told me she had one on the edge of her forest and that she could bring a chair out there and meditate with them. I saw her a month later, and as she entered the room, she glowed with happiness. She told me that meditating with the violets had brought back a childlike joy and hope that she hadn't felt in years.

Astrological association: Venus

Deities, angels, or spirit associations: Aphrodite, the fey, and angels

Meditation: Sweet little flower, bring me happiness, joy, and laughter so that I may share it with others.

Magical spell: Take dried violet leaves, rose petals, lavender, and borage leaves in equal parts and mix them together to make a tisane that will create happiness and peace, as well as fairy energy.

White Sage (*Salvia apiana*)

Common name: White prairie weed

Description: White sage is a bush that can grow 4 or 5 feet tall. It has greenish-white, lance-shaped leaves that are slightly leathery. The leaves can grow up to 3½ inches long, and each leaf has a white vein down the middle and several blunt teeth as the base. The leaves grow up the stem in alternating pairs. The flowers are white with a slight pink tinge, and each flower has five petals that are fused at the base with a small upper lip and a large lower lip. There are two long stamens that hang over the sides.

Parts used: Leaves and stalks

Caution: White sage is overharvested; please make sure that the sage that you buy is ethically sourced.

Folklore and history: The Native American folklore is different depending on the tribe. I learned from the Dakota tribe I worked with, which uses prairie sage (*Artemisia ludoviciana*), that it is used for purification of the spirit, and it is used before going into a sweat lodge or if a person is in need of healing. Since leaving Minnesota, I have started using white sage instead, as both types can be used interchangeably. I was taught to always burn the stalks when doing shamanic work because they're more powerful than the leaves.

Spiritual uses: Purification and grounding

Spiritual anecdote: I used to gather prairie sage the way I was taught, which was after it flowered and set seed. I would cut off the seeds and spread them around to help the next year's plants grow, and then I would cut the plant's stems close to the base. I would then wrap the sage with thread and let it dry in my car. I have also done this with white sage strands before the plant became scarce, and I actually had to use some freshly dried white sage one day when I went to pick up a friend who was in the process of leaving an abusive boyfriend. She was scared of him coming to find her, so after I reached her, I took a stick of white sage that was drying in my car and lit it. I then cleansed her quickly and got her and her stuff in my sage-filled car just as he drove up. I said an invisibility spell, jumped in my car, and sealed my door with sage smoke. He did not see us, and we were able to drive away quickly. One could say it was luck, but I firmly believe that an herbal wand and an invisibility spell did the trick.

Astrological association: Saturn

Deity, angel, or spirit association: White Buffalo Calf Woman

Meditation: *White sage, we honor you and the sacredness of our ancestors. Purify our hearts so that we always have the blessings of our ancestors on our journey.*

Magical spell: For home cleansing and purification, light an herbal wand made from sage and, starting at the front door, cleanse your home, walking clockwise around the inside of the home until you end up back at the front door. At the front door, make three sweeping motions to usher out any of the bad energy.

Wild Bergamot (*Monarda fistulosa*)

Common names: Bee balm, sweet leaf, and wild bee balm

Description: Wild bergamot can grow to be 3 feet tall; it is bush-like in appearance with each stem growing directly from the ground. The leaves are spear shaped with fine-toothed edges on the borders. The leaves are a pale to medium green and grow bilaterally on the stem. The stem is slightly square shaped (as the stems of most mints are) and can be anywhere from red tinged to pale green in color. This plant is prone to mildew after it flowers, so you may find the leaves covered in a white, powdery substance. The flowers are pale pink and grow at the end of each stem. The flowers have petals that are narrow and tubular in nature and appear to stick straight out from the base head of the flower. To me, the flowers look like either hair that is wild and sticking straight out or a crown sitting on the top of a head. The leaves are usually collected prior to the plant blooming.

Parts used: Leaves

Cautions: None known

Folklore and history: Most of the lore I learned about this plant came in the form of stories from my Native American teachers. Wild bergamot is a plant with a high spiritual vibration and can be used to help connect one to the ancestors. It can be mixed with tobacco and smoked to commune with the dead and can be used during a sweat to help draw the ancestors to assist with healing for a person who has dealt with a death in the family. Some Native American shamans I have met feel that it helps with walking between the worlds because its roots can go deep into the earth as its flowers rise into the sky.

Spiritual uses: Wild bergamot can be used in money and healing spells, but it can also be used for spiritual development and astral travel. This plant, to me, is very old, powerful, and spiritually advanced, and all of that should be kept in mind when using it for both magical and medicinal uses. Wild bergamot is willing to assist us in our journey toward self-discovery, and I have often meditated with this plant and have found that it makes the spiritual path easier to tread. It gently shows you the way and gives you new insights into where you need to journey next. I usually have people drink a tea or a tincture containing it, and I have given wild bergamot tea to people who lacked direction (in the mundane and spiritual world). The herbal tea, along with meditation, helped them embark on the proper path. I also use it in bags with mugwort and blue vervain and stuff it under pillows to use during dream time to move into the other worlds. I have also used it to help regrow hair, which can be quite magical in someone with long-term hair loss.

Spiritual anecdote: I once met a man who was a friend of a friend, and when he looked at me, I saw an emptiness in his soul. To me, this indicated that part of his soul was lost in the other world. I talked to him for a while and found out that his mom died while giving birth to him and that he almost died during the birthing time. He also told me that he had never felt whole and that he felt like there was this deep chasm. Sometimes he wished he could dive into it and disappear. I asked him if he wanted to be whole, and he said that he didn't know what "whole" meant and confessed that he felt like part of him was taken when his mother died. He wanted to feel better, but he did not know how. I had him come to my office. First, I did a medicinal consult with him but then took him to my ritual space to cleanse him and help him reconnect with the lost parts of his soul. One of the herbs I used to help him reconnect was wild bergamot. I made him an herbal tea to drink before the journey, and then I put it in a bag for him to carry with him.

Astrological association: Venus

Deities, angels, or spirit associations: Hera, Aphrodite, and ancestors

Meditation: Ancient plant spirit, guide me on this path. Light the way so that I may see which way to walk; help me brighten the darkest corners.

Magical spell: Take wild bergamot, mix in equal parts mugwort and vervain, and drink it as a tisane before doing astral travel. It will not only relax you and open you for travel, but it will help make the journey easier, as you will be a little stronger in the other worlds as you journey.

Wild Carrot (*Daucus carota*)

Common names: Queen Anne's lace, bird's nest, and bee's nest

Description: Wild carrot starts blooming around midsummer in North America. The plant is often found along roadsides, in ditches, and in waste areas, and it is easily identified by its flower head, which is white and lacy with a red flower in the center. In full bloom it has multiple small, white brackets that form this flat umbrella-type flower head. The leaves are feathery and grow in alternate pairs. Wild carrot is a biennial plant, which blooms and sets seed in its second year. When the flowers are getting past their prime, they draw together to form a head-shaped cup. At this point the seeds have formed and are ripe for picking. The seeds are small, pointed, and able to penetrate even the poorest soils. The plant is related to the domesticated carrot, but unlike the carrot we are used to seeing in stores, it has a taproot that is white and thin that goes deep into the earth.

Parts used: Leaves and roots

Caution: Do not ingest if pregnant or breastfeeding.

Folklore and history: Legends say that the red flower in the center of the flower head came from a drop of blood from Queen Anne's finger. It is said that she was trying to conceive the next heir to the throne by using Witchcraft and that the drop of her blood was an ingredient that bound the spell. In the time of Dioscorides, the seeds were used to protect against the bites of venomous beasts.

Spiritual uses: Lust magic, fertility, strength, and helping someone become more grounded; magically, there has not been much written about the use of wild carrot, but by using the doctrine of signatures, we can determine the plant's magical purposes. When I think about wild carrot, several things come to mind. First of all, I think of the plant's determination. This plant can seed in most types of soil, even the hardest of clay, indicating fertility, strength, and determination. When I see the closed seed head, I think it looks like a head that is separated from its body by a series of feathery leaves. This, to me, indicates a separation of the head from the needs of the body, which means the plant can help someone who is either lost in the spirit world or disassociated from their body—either from force or by choice. A tincture of both the flower head and the root helps bring a person who's too astral/unbalanced to a more balanced perspective. The seeds can also be added to fertility-enhancing incense; I like to mix them with mints and poppy seeds.

Spiritual anecdote: I had a friend who was spacey—and not in the normal way. She was obsessed with space and thought she was an alien. She didn't think she was abducted, but she did believe she was put here to study humans. She also tripped over almost everything in her path, which I learned from my Native American teachers means that the spirit is not connected to the earth. She was obsessed, and she realized this, so she came to me to see if I could ground her a bit. I taught her how to ground using common techniques, and then I tried a few herbs on her, including wood betony and wild carrot. I was expecting the wood betony to be a better choice, but the wild carrot tested better. Within the first week of taking a tincture of wild carrot, she felt much more stable, and I noticed right away that she was not looking up at the stars as much. She also stopped tripping over every little rock in her path. She still thought that she was an alien, but that is what made her such an interesting person.

Astrological association: Mars

Deities, angels, or spirit associations: Artemis and Cerridwen

Meditation: *Root so deep and strong, help me achieve my desires; help me reach my goals.*

Magical spell: Dig up a wild carrot root and clean it off. While chanting the plant's meditation, concentrate on what your greatest desire is. Wrap the root in red thread and place it under your pillow during the full moon. You should then dream of how to obtain your goal.

Wild Geranium (*Geranium maculatum*)

Common names: Alum root, cranesbill, spotted cranesbill, wild cranesbill, storksbill, chocolate flower, crowfoot, dovefoot, and shameface

Description: Wild geranium grows up to 2 feet tall and has dark green, deeply serrated leaves that develop on individual stalks that rise out of the ground. This particular species of wild geranium has seven lobes on each leaf. The individual lobes are cut almost to the bottom center of each leaf, and each lobe has teeth surrounding it. The purplish flowers, which bloom in early June, have five petals with long stigmas. These long stigmas ripen to form long, thin seedpods, which resemble crane bills.

Parts used: Roots

Cautions: None known

Folklore and history: While this herb is mentioned in M. Grieve's *A Modern Herbal, King's American Dispensatory*, and John Scudder's *Specific Medication and Specific Medicines*, there isn't a lot of folklore written about it. It is a plant indigenous to the United States and is a powerful astringent for hemorrhoids and bowel issues. I learned about it from my Native American teachers and from using it in my practice.

Spiritual uses: In studying this plant for magical use, it became apparent quite quickly that this was not your garden-variety magical plant. The spirit of wild geranium is very old, and it told me tales of having deep roots that extend to the center of the earth. These roots are able to draw the very essence of life and bring it back to us. When I was talking to and meditating with the wild geranium, it also told me the story of when it was first used. A young man, who was going into battle for the first time, had a vision of this plant saving his life during the next day's skirmish. So, the young man took a leaf of the plant with him. He only received a small wound during the fight, and he put the leaf on it as the spirit of the plant had instructed him to do. That night the young man started having nightmares about the battle and was unable to sleep. The next morning, he told a village elder about his plant vision and the disturbing thoughts and nightmares. The elder took some of the plant leaves and brewed him an herbal tea and told him to drink it every day until the nightmares subsided. The young man did as he was instructed, and not only did the nightmares subside, but he gained the favor of the plant spirits and became a great healer.

So, what does all of this tell us about wild geranium's magical uses? On the simplest level, this plant is a great protector and can be carried when extra protection is needed, especially when you feel like you must fight to win. It is also a plant that is willing to share great knowledge of new skills and help develop latent talents. Wild geranium can also be used to heal people or situations on both the mundane and spiritual levels so that new growth can take place. This is one of the herbs that I add to bags for people who are going through changes so quickly that they feel like their heads are spinning and they're out of control. It helps center, strengthen, and put people on the right path. This herb can be used for protection, courage, and forging new paths.

Spiritual anecdote: I had a student who was a great healer but lacked the confidence to start a practice and felt like she was not good enough to charge people money for her services. I dug a root of wild geranium out of my forest and made a bag for her that included the root, some tiger-eye, rose quartz, and citrine. I had her carry it in her purse and, when she was selling at the farmer's market, in her money bag. Her first client walked right up to her at a farmers' market about a week after I made the bag for her and asked her if she knew anything about arthritis, and she said, "Why yes, I do." She then got bolder and started writing for a local natural magazine. Within a year, she had a full practice with clients.

Astrological association: Mars

Deities, angels, or spirit associations: Hecate and Cernunnos

Meditation: Sweet, innocent plant, assist me with your virtues to help me (insert need).

Magical spell: Dig up a wild geranium root under a full moon or buy dried root at the store. Put the root in a bag (use a red bag if you are trying to attract love and green if you want to have more money) along with the appropriate stones, and chant the above meditation over it three times every day from full moon to full moon.

Wild Lettuce (*Lactuca virosa*)

Common names: Acrid lettuce, poor man's opium, bitter lettuce, opium lettuce, poison lettuce, and great lettuce

Description: Wild lettuce is a biennial plant that has a dark brown taproot and a light green stem that is smooth with a light reddish-purple flush. The plant can grow up to 6½ feet tall, and its large leaves grow alternately up the stem. These leaves are bright green, deeply lobed, and serrated along the edges. They wrap slightly around the stem and are easily identified by the whitish midvein down the center. The vein is raised on both the top and the bottom of the leaf. On the bottom, there are small hairs on the rib called trichomes. The plant is also easily identified by a white sap that comes from the stems or leaves when cut or ripped. The flowers grow from small stems that develop at the top of the plant. The flowers are small and yellow with eight to twelve flat-edged petals and a simple double-headed stamen. The seeds are small, black, and oval in shape. They have a wing at one end that is attached to a white, fluffy aerial that allows transport on the wind.

Parts used: Leaves and white sap

Cautions: Do not use in large amounts as it will make you fall asleep; do not use before you drive or use machinery.

Folklore and history: Wild lettuce is a native European plant that was brought to the United States by immigrants. According to M. Grieve, author of *A Modern Herbal*, King Augustus was once very ill and wild lettuce was given to help cure him. He was so happy with the results he set up an altar to it in his home and gave it a place of honor in his healer's apothecary. Since the Middle Ages, wild lettuce, also called wild opium, has been used as an opium substitute or as an additive to the drug to extend it. It has been used to relieve pain externally and used internally as a hypnotic.

Spiritual uses: Trance work, meditation, entering hypnotic states, improving creativity, and relieving pain; wild lettuce is a great herb to use to get you in a relaxed state before you do any kind of magical work. It is a little bitter, so if you drink it as a tisane, make sure to add herbs that have a pungent or sweet flavor to counteract it. I usually mix it with peppermint or chamomile. Even a small amount will help you get into a trance state, which it does by relaxing you and opening the mind. If too much is used, it will just make you sleepy. I have heard stories of many people overusing this herb, thinking that it will be a drug substitute, and while it does have a mild effect, it is not that strong.

Spiritual anecdote: I have a friend, whom I'll call Bob, who is a very scholarly ceremonial magician. Bob was having issues relaxing during his rituals, and he felt like if he relaxed just a little bit he would have better luck calling spirits and demons into his circle. His goal in contacting these entities was to gain knowledge of lost magical arts, so I offered a formula of wild lettuce, chamomile, and peppermint in equal parts for him to drink before he started his magical workings. He decided to make an entire coffee pot of the blend instead of the cup I suggested and drank it before entering his circle. This large amount made Bob slightly sleepy during the ritual, but he did report seeing some apparition come through, which gave him some information that he wasn't expecting. I explained to him that just a cup of this blend would have worked just as well, and he started adding it to his pre-ritual routine because it worked so well.

Astrological association: Moon

Deities, angels, or spirit associations: Hypnos, Nyx, and Artemis

Meditation: Herb of grace, help me get into a state of relaxation, let my mind see the things that are hidden in the dark, and let me hear wisdom on my journey.

Magical spell: Before a ritual, take 1 teaspoon of wild lettuce, 1 tablespoon of peppermint leaf, and 1 teaspoon of blue vervain. Mix the herbs together, put 1 tablespoon in a muslin tea bag, pour hot (but not boiling) water over the herbs, and let them steep for ten minutes. Drink this before ritual or before doing any magical work where you need to go into a trance or do deep magical work.

Wild Yam (*Dioscorea villosa*)

Common names: Dioscorea, colicroot, and rheumatism root

Description: The wild yam had its beginning in tropical regions, but it is easily grown in subtropical to tropic regions. In fact, you can often find the plant in the wild in North and Central America if you know what to look for. It is a vining plant with heart-shaped, glossy leaves that grow in pairs on a delicate reddish stem. It has small, unremarkable greenish-white flowers that shoot off joints on the stem, often resembling shooting stars. The plant dies back in the fall and returns in the spring. The part that is used is the fleshy rhizome, which should be dug up in the fall.

Parts used: Roots and rhizomes

Cautions: Do not ingest if pregnant or nursing.

Folklore and history: Not a lot of magical lore has been written about wild yam in English, but if you look at its doctrine of signatures, you can see what it can be used for. It has heart-shaped leaves, which indicate love. The stems are red tinged, which can indicate a connection to blood vessels, but it can also indicate a connection to the other world. The flowers are small and whitish green, and there are both male and female flowers on the same plant. These signatures can indicate increased sexuality or love, as well as general healing. Considering that the plant is used for menopausal woman to balance hormones, I can see that it can be used to restore sexuality and balance. One of the few folk uses I've learned about was a Mexican custom that includes mashing the fresh rhizome with honey and cornmeal and serving it to a prospective husband in order to bind the marriage contract before he develops eyes for another.

Spiritual uses: Fertility, love magic, creating rainstorms, and increasing strength when dealing with emotionally taxing situations; in order to increase one's inner strength during emotional times, take the root of wild yam with you whenever you go somewhere that may bring you internal conflict. To attract a romantic partner, cut a piece of the root and hang it around your neck. I have used it to increase sexuality in people, giving it as a tisane to people who've lost their sexual desire due to menopause, and I have used it in bags for people to increase sexuality in long-term relationships—it helps bring back the spark. I wouldn't call this an herb of lust. Instead, I would say it's an herb to balance sexual desire. I have also used it in helping people who are extremely stressed get through a hard time. Another thing I have used it for is as a pathway toward the other worlds. The leaves and stems in an incense mixed with mugwort and angelica can help with traveling to other dimensions.

Spiritual anecdote: I had a husband and wife as my clients, and they came to me for some medical issues. One of the things I ask about in my consults is sexuality. Well, they just laughed and said that they had become "friends" and were no longer having intercourse. So, I created blends for them to balance out their medical issues, and I also gave them each a small wild yam root to carry with them. I told them to hold it in their hand once a day while thinking about the other person. At their next visit, they told me they had rekindled their romantic relationship.

Astrological association: Mercury

Deities, angels, or spirit associations: Aphrodite and Chimalma

Meditation: Plant of the air, root of the earth, help me balance between the worlds.

Magical spells: For romance, take a piece of the root and carry it and think about your love daily. For travel between the worlds, take the stem and burn it in incense or carry it to help you obtain access to other worlds.

Wood Sorrel (*Oxalis acetosella*)

Common names: Greensauce, sour grabs, sour sauce, cuckoo sorrel, and sorrow dock

Description: Wood sorrel grows to be around 5 inches tall, and there are two colors that the leaves of the plant can come in: red and green. Leaf shape and the basic flower structure are the same regardless of color. Each leaf has three lobes, and each of these lobes is divided in half by a center vein, which makes the lobes look like hearts. The lobes are all connected at the bottom of the leaf. The leaves have a distinct lemon taste. The red wood sorrel flower is lilac in color, while the flowers on the green wood sorrel are white with pale purple veins. Both the leaves and the flowers come from the ends of delicate-looking stems, and both are open during the day but close at night, during rainstorms, and when touched. Wood sorrel spreads by both seeds and creeping roots, even though it is not invasive. It flowers continuously from late spring to early fall and is edible the entire time.

Parts used: Leaves

Cautions: Wood sorrel is high in oxalic acid and should not be ingested by people who have a history of kidney stones; consume drinks made from the plant only occasionally due to the oxalic acid.

Folklore and history: This herb has been used as a food by Europeans for hundreds of years, and small children in England collected the herb and sucked on the stems to extract the tartness.

Spiritual uses: Wood sorrel has not really been explored in many of the older occult herbals, but it still can be used magically. Using the doctrine of signatures, I can see this herb to be goddess-oriented due to its triple leaf, sensitive nature, and delicate flower. The herb is very cooling, even though it has a tart taste to it, so one could use this herb to magically cool down angry or bitter situations. It could also be used to increase psychic abilities or sensitivity in general. I have used wood sorrel in an incense as a purification aid along with frankincense and cedar; the wood sorrel added a pleasing bite to the blend and rounded out the incense quite nicely. I have also used it in a tea blend to increase psychic abilities.

Spiritual anecdote: I had a spiritual student who was having issues developing her psychic abilities. She could not tolerate the usual mugwort, so I went out in my garden, picked some wood sorrel, and made her an herbal tea with it before we started practicing reading tarot cards. It helped open the way for the imagery to come through, and she made a beverage with this herb every time she was doing deep work with her tarot cards until she didn't need it anymore.

Astrological association: Venus

Deities, angels, or spirit associations: Brigid and Hecate

Meditation: Little plant that holds so much life, help me see clearly. Help me see what is hidden.

Magical spells: Take a little of the fresh plant and make a tea with it to drink before doing divination, or take a bit of the dried plant and add it to a sleep pillow alongside mugwort to increase dream time visions.

Wormwood (*Artemisia absinthium*)

Common names: Artemisia, wermout, wormod, and green ginger

Description: Wormwood is a small, shrubby bush, rarely growing more than 3 feet tall. The stems come directly from the ground and are flexible and nonwoody. The 3- to 5-inch leaves, which are greenish gray on the top and white on the bottom, grow spirally around the stems. They are very fine, hairy, yielding to the touch, and very aromatic. The plant's flowers grow at the end of the stems. They are small, light yellow, and discoid, meaning they have no petals.

Parts used: Leaves

Cautions: Be careful when using alongside medications; it can have side effects with certain antidepressants and other medications.

Folklore and history: Wormwood's Latin name, *Artemisia*, comes from the goddess Artemis. M. Grieve, in *A Modern Herbal*, writes that in a translation of Apuleius's *Herbarium* that "Diana did find them and delivered their powers and leechdom [remedy] to Chiron the Centaur, who first from these Worts [plant] set forth a leechdom, and he named these worts from the name of Diana, Artemis." There are several Victorian love spells that used wormwood to help a person see their future love in their dreams. In one, wormwood was put under a person's pillow. In another, it was mixed with other herbs, put it in honey, and eaten before going to bed. Wormwood is an herb that can help with divination, which is why the Victorians used it. They mixed it with honey because it is a very bitter herb.

Spiritual uses: Divination, love, opening doorways, and communicating with the fey

Spiritual anecdote: I use wormwood in ritual incense, and when it is used with frankincense, it can be a powerful trance inducer. One of the interesting things that happens when using it during outdoor rituals is that members of the fey come to join the festivities. I once did a ritual at a campground with my group, and as I went into the forest to leave offerings, I heard the wind whisper that it liked the scent in the air. I then saw a tree spirit in the distance. I turned around to walk out of the space and discovered that the trees had changed and the rock that marked the exit was gone. I think that the incense woke something up in the forest, and whoever it was watched our ritual.

Astrological association: Mars

Deities, angels, or spirit associations: Diana, Artemis, plant spirits, and the fey

Meditation: *Wormwood, O silvery mound, help me open the doorways to get me to the other worlds.*

Magical spell: Take 1 part wormwood, 1 part vervain, 1 part dandelion leaf, and 1 part frankincense and mix them together. Burn the mix as incense while saying the plant's meditation and envisioning traveling to other worlds or dimensions.

Yarrow (*Achilla millefolium*)

Common names: Stanch grass, bloodwort, dog daisy, knight's balm, Devil's nettle, and soldier's woundwort

Description: Yarrow is easily identified. In midsummer the plant reaches a height of up to 3 feet, and its leaves are feather- or fernlike, silvery green in color, and highly fragrant. Yarrow flowers from June until October, usually in sunny and flat areas, and its small, daisylike flowers are often white or pinkish and develop in large, flat clusters. It is best to collect it in July—once the flowers have opened.

Parts used: Flowers and leaves

Cautions: None known

Folklore and history: Yarrow is one of the oldest plants used medicinally and magically. In northern Iraq, fossilized yarrow has been found in a Neanderthal burial cave, and carbon dating of this material puts it at more than sixty thousand years old. It has been recorded by E. A. Wallis Budge that yarrow was used in ancient Egypt and medicinally in India for more than five thousand years. The original I Ching divining tool was several stripped and dried yarrow stems.

In Greek mythology it was said that Chiron, the eldest in a race of centaurs and the teacher of Asclepius, Hercules, and Achilles, imparted the knowledge of yarrow's healing properties to Achilles before he went into battle. As the myth goes, Achilles covered himself in yarrow everywhere except his heel, which is the only place an arrow was able to pierce him.

The Saxons wore charms stuffed with yarrow to protect them against highway robbers, firestorms, and blindness, and in France it became one of the herbs burned in the bonfires to celebrate Saint John's day and Midsummer Eve and for protection against harm. Yarrow has been the subject of many love and healing spells, and a folk incantation recited in England says:

> *There's a crying at my window and a hand upon my door,*
> *and a stir among the yarrow that's fading on the floor.*

The voice cries at my window, the hand on my door beats on,
but if I heed and answer them, sure hand and voice are gone.

In Victorian times, young girls used yarrow in a spell to see the great love in their future, saying:

Thou pretty herb of Venus' tree,
thy true name is yarrow.
Now who my bosom love must be
pray tell thou me tomorrow.

Those words were said three times before going to sleep on a small pillow filled with yarrow.

Spiritual uses: Yarrow has many magical virtues, which include courage, love, purification, protection from fires or thieves, and increasing psychic abilities. The flowers can be made into an herbal tea to improve psychic abilities, and a bunch of yarrow hung over the bed will ensure love for seven years. A sprig of yarrow on each windowsill and under the doormat of your home will prevent anyone from entering that wishes to do you harm and prevent fires. When worn, yarrow will protect you from harm, and when carried it will give courage. I personally put sprigs of yarrow in every windowsill and at each door to prevent harm from coming across those boundaries. I also have a small bundle in my car to keep me safe when driving.

Spiritual anecdote: I once had a student who had to give her doctoral dissertation, and she was scared out of her wits. I gave her a sprig of yarrow to carry into the dissertation for courage and to prevent someone on the dissertation committee from causing her added stress. She was easily able to defend her dissertation, and the professor she was most afraid of was not even there.

Astrological association: Venus

Deities, angels, or spirit associations: Archangels, centaurs, Aphrodite, and Queen of the Fairies

Meditation: *Yarrow, sweet yarrow, protect me from harm and make me stronger so that I can stay steadfast on my path.*

Magic spell: Take a few sprigs of yarrow, tie them together with red thread, and hang them from each window to protect your home from harm. To get the best results, say the plant's meditation while wrapping the yarrow.

Yew (*Taxus baccata*)

Common names: Common yew, English yew, and European yew

Description: The yew tree is a member of the conifer family and can grow up to 65 feet tall with a thick trunk that can reach up to 13 feet wide. The dark brown outer bark is thin and easily flakes off; the inner bark is reddish brown. When looking at older yew trees, you will see exposed roots at the base of the trunks. The stems of the tree grow up the trunk in an alternating pattern. The leaves are approximately 1½ inches long, flat, short, dark green, and arranged in a spiral pattern around the stems. Since yews are conifers, they do not produce flowers. Instead, they produce cones that are green when unripe but bright red when mature. The seeds are dark brown, flattish on one end, and pointed on the other. The trees are dioecious but can be both male and female at the same time or switch from one sex to the other. Scientists still do not understand the triggers that cause these changes to happen.

Parts used: Berries

Cautions: Yew is toxic; do not take internally and do not burn in incense. Some people are very sensitive to the toxins. Even touching the leaves can cause a reaction.

Folklore and history: The yew tree is poisonous, and only the cones can be safely used. It was often planted in churchyards and graveyards too. In fact, the oldest known yew tree is in a churchyard in the Scottish village of Fortingall. It is estimated to be two thousand to three thousand years old. Some yew trees have holes in the trunks so large they can be walked through, and in some cases, a few trees have been made into small rooms in churches. Some people think yew trees were planted near churches and graveyards to help cover up the smell of decay, but it might have been a holdover from the Gauls or Druids, who planted the trees to give spirits a gateway into the underworld. It is said that the yew is an underworld tree and used by Hecate.

Yew is featured several times in Shakespeare's plays, and one of my favorite mentions is in act 4, scene 1 of Macbeth, when the three witches are mixing their brew. Part of their chant is "Slips of Yew slivered in the moon's eclipse."

Spiritual uses: Because it is toxic, yew is best grown as an outdoor tree and dedicated as an underworld portal for spirits. It should not be used in ritual.

Spiritual anecdote: The college I went to was located next to a graveyard that was more than one hundred years old, and the entry to the graveyard had a row of six yews on each side. Part of my group's annual Halloween ritual practice was to go through the graveyards, clean off headstones that had been neglected, and leave flowers on the graves. One Halloween a group of us were walking out of the graveyard, and we noticed a hole tunneled under one of the old yews. As we drew closer, we noticed what looked like smoke or steam coming from it. All of a sudden, a rabbit ran out of the hole and gave us such a fright we ran out of the graveyard. A few days later, I went back to the graveyard and looked at the yew where the hole had been—and there was no hole! In fact, there was no evidence that a hole had ever been there. I then called one of the other people who had been there that night and had them come check. They couldn't find a hole either. We asked the caretaker of the graveyard about it later that year, and he said that we should stay away from those old yews because that was where the Devil came out to grab souls and drag them down to hell with him. Needless to say, we didn't go back to that graveyard that close to Halloween again.

I work with the spirit of the tree rather than harvest or use the plant itself due to its toxicity. I often talk to this spirit when someone has died, and I ask it to provide a doorway to allow them to pass into the other world.

Astrological association: Saturn

Deity, angel, or spirit association: Hecate

Meditation: *Sacred yew, gateway to the underworld, I respect your power over death and as a gateway to the underworld. Please help* (insert name) *to pass into the other world safely.*

Magical spell: When someone has died and you want to help their soul transition, take a branch of yew and say the plant's meditation three times before burying it in the earth.

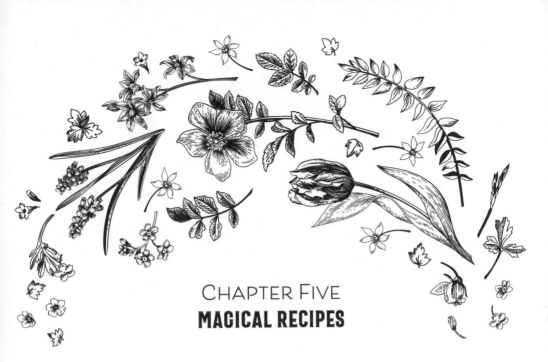

CHAPTER FIVE
MAGICAL RECIPES

These are recipes that I have used in my practice. If you do not have one of the ingredients listed in a recipe, look at the appendix to find a plant that meets your need and you also have access to. You can then replace the ingredient you don't have with it. If you need a reminder on how to make teas, tisanes, salves, or oils, please refer to chapter 3, which gives detailed instructions on how to make these items.

The amounts needed for each incense and tea recipe are written in parts, which is a volume measurement. If you have a teaspoon of each herb, that is considered a part for that formula. If you have a cup of each herb, that is also considered a part for that formula. I structured the recipes this way because an ounce (weight measurement) of one herb is not equal in volume to another herb. For example, 1 ounce of calendula will fill 2 cups, whereas 1 ounce of frankincense will only be ½ cup. The amounts needed for the essential oils are written in drops and cups, which are also volume measurements; some of the infused oils have the dried herbs written in parts.

Incense

Most of these incense recipes can be mixed up ahead of time and then placed directly on charcoals to burn. Store them in glass jars to maintain freshness.

Incense Blends for the Fey, Spirits, and Demons

These incense blends will be helpful to attract or repel the fey, spirits, or demons. Be aware that some of the banishing recipes have strong herbs in them, and it is advisable to open windows to increase ventilation when burning them.

Incense to Call the Fey

- 1 part fern leaf
- 1 part violet leaf
- 1 part frankincense
- 1 part lilac flowers

Grind ingredients together until finely powdered and burn on a charcoal.

Incense to Get Rid of Unwanted Fey

- 1 part yellow dock root
- 1 part myrrh
- 1 pinch asafetida

Grind ingredients together until finely powdered and burn on a charcoal.

Incense to Get Rid of Psychic Vampires

- 1 part garlic powder
- 1 pinch asafetida
- 1 part dried hyacinth flowers

Grind ingredients together until finely powdered and burn on a charcoal.

Spirit Be-Gone Incense

- 1 part basil
- 1 part yarrow
- 1 part myrrh

Grind ingredients together until finely powdered and burn on a charcoal.

Incense to Get Rid of Demons

- 1 part garlic powder
- ½ part asafetida
- 1 part frankincense
- 1 part myrrh
- 1 part benzoin
- 1 part rosemary
- 3 drops of holy water
- 3 drops of red wine (representing the blood of Jesus)

Grind ingredients together until finely powdered; open windows before burning on a charcoal.

Incense Blends for Love

These blends are for all stages of love, including lust. There's a true love recipe, which can also be used to promote self-love, and a long-term love recipe.

Keep Love Strong Incense

- 1 part rose petals
- 1 part lavender
- 1 part yarrow

Grind ingredients together until finely powdered and burn on a charcoal.

True Love Incense

- 1 part yarrow
- 1 part pennyroyal
- 1 part frankincense
- 2 drops of rose geranium essential oil

Grind ingredients together until finely powdered and burn on a charcoal.

Lust Incense

- 1 part dragon's blood (powdered)
- 1 part rose petals
- 1 part damiana

Grind ingredients together until finely powdered and burn on a charcoal.

Incense Blends to Increase Luck

These incense recipes are to increase your luck in love, money, or anything else you want to improve your luck with.

Incense to Increase Your Luck

- 1 part holly leaves
- 1 part wood rose
- 1 part fern leaves
- ½ part allspice (ground)

Grind the ingredients together while concentrating on your intent. Burn on a charcoal.

Incense to Increase Your Luck #2

- 1 part lemon balm
- 1 part basil
- 1 part cedar
- 1 part daffodil flower

Grind each ingredient separately, and then mix them with your intention firmly in your mind. Burn on a charcoal.

Incense Blends to Protect against Negative Influences

These blends are used to clear a space or person of negativity or negative influences.

Protection from Negative Influences

- 1 part white sage
- 1 part lavender flowers
- 1 part sweetgrass

Grind ingredients together until finely powdered. Burn on a charcoal or sprinkle around a space.

Reversing Negativity Incense
- 1 part vervain
- 1 part frankincense
- 1 part garden sage
- 1 part basil

Grind ingredients together and burn on a charcoal. It is best to burn this incense outdoors.

Peaceful Home Incense
- 1 part chamomile flowers
- 1 part meadowsweet leaves
- 1 part lavender flowers
- 1 part pennyroyal herb

Mix ingredients and burn on coals to promote a peaceful and loving environment.

Prosperity Incense Blends
These blends are to increase the amount of money or prosperity in your life.

Fast-Money Incense
- 1 part basil
- 1 part galangal root
- 1 part lavender

Grind all the ingredients together while concentrating on your intent. Burn on a charcoal.

Prosperity Incense
- 1 part ground ivy
- 1 part basil
- ½ part poppy seeds
- ½ part copal

Powder all ingredients and mix them together with your intent firmly in mind. Burn the mixture on charcoals.

Protection Incense Blends

These blends will help protect you or your home from harm.

Protection against Personal Harm Incense

- 1 part prickly ash bark
- 1 part myrrh
- 1 part agrimony
- 1 part lady's mantle

Grind all ingredients together while concentrating on your goal. Burn the incense on an incense charcoal.

Protection against Witchcraft

- 1 part vervain
- 1 part angelica root
- 1 part dragon's blood

Grind all ingredients together while concentrating on your goal. Burn the incense on an incense charcoal.

Home Protection Incense Blend

- 1 part frankincense
- 1 part oak wood
- 1 part lavender
- Pinch of salt

Grind all ingredients together while concentrating on your goal. Burn the incense on an incense charcoal.

Purification Incense Blends

These blends are used to purify a space or a person.

Wood Betony Purification Incense

- 1 part wood betony leaves (powdered)
- 1 part frankincense (powdered)
- ½ part sandalwood (powdered)
- ½ part cedarwood (powdered)

Mix the ingredients together while concentrating on the intention of purification. Burn on a charcoal.

Three Goddesses Purification Incense
- 1 part frankincense
- 1 part benzoin
- 1 part myrrh

Mix the ingredients together while concentrating on the intention of purification. Burn on a charcoal.

Rue Purification Incense
- 1 part rue leaves
- 1 part frankincense
- 1 part cedar wood
- 1 part rosemary

Grind the ingredients individually until powdered, and then mix them together while focusing on your goal. Burn the mixture on a charcoal. This incense is especially good for pre-ritual purification.

Ritual Incense Blends
These incense blends are to be used in rituals to help you connect with the Divine.

Flying Incense
- ¼ part nightshade leaf (belladonna or black nightshade)
- 1 part camphor
- 1 part blue vervain
- 1 part mugwort

While wearing gloves, grind each ingredient individually, and then blend them together while concentrating on your goal. Burn on charcoal to help with astral travel and intense ritual magic. Use this in small amounts and in a well-ventilated area. *CAUTION: This formula is toxic in large amounts.*

Initiation Incense

- 1 part rose petals
- 1 part oakmoss
- 1 part blue vervain
- ½ part pine needles or bark
- ½ part rowan leaves
- ½ part yarrow flowers

Grind ingredients together until finely powdered and burn on a charcoal.

Scrying Incense Blends

These incense blends will help with divination, scrying, or psychic work.

Divination Incense

- 1 part mugwort
- 1 part blue vervain
- 1 part orris root

Grind the ingredients together and burn the mixture on a charcoal with your intent firmly in mind.

Tarot Reading Incense

- 1 part lavender flowers
- 1 part clary sage
- 1 part peppermint
- 1 part wormwood

Grind the ingredients individually and blend them together. Burn the combination on a charcoal as you do tarot readings.

Psychic Development Incense

- 1 part calendula
- 1 part yarrow
- 1 part mugwort

Grind the ingredients individually and blend them together. Put the combination on a charcoal with your intent firmly in mind.

Oils and Perfumes

Oils and perfumes are wonderful magical tools that can be mixed ahead of time and put in dark glass jars to keep fresh for years.

Infused Oils

Infuse the herbs in the oils for a simple way to make your own natural spiritual perfumes and anointing oils.

Infused Calendula Flower Oil

- ½ ounce of dried calendula flowers
- 2 cups of almond oil

Place the dried flowers and oil in a pot that is in another pot filled at least a quarter of the way full of water (double boiler method) on your stove top. Turn the heat on low and simmer for three to four hours while stirring frequently to avoid burning. The oil should turn golden yellow in color when it is finished. Once the oil has cooled, strain the flowers from the oil and store the oil in a dark-colored jar.

Daisy-Infused Oil

- 4 cups of fresh daisy heads
- 2 cups of almond oil

Gather the daisies during the day, after the sun has dried off the morning dew, and dehydrate them in an oven or dehydrator. (If you do not have access to fresh daisies, you can use 2 cups of dried daisies; it takes about 4 cups of fresh daisies to get 2 cups of dried daisies.) Make sure they are fully dried, and add 1 cup of them to a Mason jar. Add the oil to the jar, seal it, and put it in a sunny window for three weeks. After three weeks, strain the herbs and the remaining cup of dried daisies. Steep for another three weeks. After six weeks have passed, strain and store the oil in a dark-colored jar. Use the oil as a rub for bruises and arthritis as well as to promote happiness.

Dragon's Blood Oil

- 4 ounces of dragon's blood resin
- 2 cups of oil
- 20 drops of scented oil of your choice

Heat the oil in a pot on your stove top's lowest setting and add resin to the oil. Stir the mixture frequently to avoid burning. Bring it to a simmer and cook until the resin is melted into the oil and the oil is the color of blood. There is a dragon's blood fragrance oil that you can add to your blend, if you choose, or you could use any oil that helps you strengthen the magical work you will be doing. Once the scented oil has been mixed in, cool and store the oil in a dark-colored jar. Use it to anoint tools for protection or in formulas to increase the strength of the spell.

Egyptian Perfume Oil

- 50 drops of myrrh oil
- 50 drops of sandalwood oil
- 25 drops of frankincense oil
- 25 drops of cardamom oil
- 10 drops of vetiver oil
- 10 strands of saffron
- 50 drops of fine red wine
- 1 cup of sweet almond oil

In a saucepan, simmer the saffron and wine in almond oil on low until the saffron has imparted a golden-red color to the oil and the wine has evaporated. Take the oil off the heat, let the oil cool, then strain out the saffron. Once cooled, add the essential oils. Store in a dark-colored jar.

Oil to Build Inner Strength

- 2 cups of oil
- 1 part cleavers
- 1 part mugwort
- 1 part yarrow
- 20 drops of myrrh essential oil
- 20 drops of dragon's blood oil

Add the herbs to 2 cups of oil in a saucepot and simmer on low for one to two hours on your stove top. Let the oil cool, then remove the herbs and strain the oil of particles.

Money-Attracting Oil
- 2 cups of oil
- 1 cup of pine needles
- ½ cup of dried basil leaves dried
- ¼ cup of galangal root
- 20 drops of patchouli oil
- Twenty-dollar bill
- Rubber band

Mix all of the ingredients in a glass Mason jar during a full moon while concentrating on your intention. Seal the jar and wrap the twenty-dollar bill around it, securing it with the rubber band. Place the jar under the light of the moon for thirty days. After thirty days, strain the herbs from the oil blend. Rub a bit of the oil on the twenty-dollar bill and spend it. Store the rest of the oil in a cool, dark place. Put a small amount of oil on money or dab some on your wallet to encourage money to come your way.

Ritual Anointing Oil
- 2 cups of dragon's blood infused oil (see the Dragon's Blood Oil recipe)
- 20 drops of benzoin essential oil
- 20 drops of frankincense essential oil
- 20 drops of myrrh essential oil
- 2 drops of cinnamon essential oil

Mix all of these ingredients together in a Mason jar. Seal the jar and store it in a cool, dark place. This oil can be used to anoint people or sacred tools prior to ritual; it both purifies and amplifies energies.

Saint John's Wort Oil

- 2 cups of fresh Saint John's wort flowers
- 2 cups of olive oil

Put flowers in a glass container and add the oil. Let the mixture sit in the sun for six weeks, or until the oil is a deep red. I use Saint John's wort oil for protection and healing.

Peppermint Cleanse and Protection Oil

- 1 part peppermint
- 1 part rosemary
- 1 part lemon peel
- 20 drops of frankincense oil
- 2 cups of oil
- 2 tablespoons of sea salt

Steep all of the ingredients except for the salt together for at least two hours. Let the oil cool, and then strain the herbs and add the salt.

This oil blend is specifically used to cleanse non-metal tools and magical objects after they have been used in open ritual. I also rub it on my hands after open ritual to make sure I don't pick up any unwanted energies.

Vervain-Infused Divination Oil

- 1 part dried vervain
- 1 cup of almond oil
- 10 drops of clary sage essential oil
- 10 drops of wormwood essential oil

Place the vervain and oil in a pot and place that pot in another pot filled at least a quarter of the way full with water (double boiler method). Turn the heat on low and simmer for three to four hours while stirring frequently to avoid burning. Once the oil has been heated for three to four hours, strain the plant from the oil, add the essential oils, and store the oil in a dark-colored jar. This oil can be used for initiation rituals or to assist with divination.

Tisanes

Teas can be taken internally, placed into a bath, or sprinkled around an area. They are best prepared with the freshest herbs possible and stored in glass containers in a dark closet. For most teas, use 1 teaspoon of herb for each cup of water and steep for ten minutes. Infusions are made with leaves and flowers, and decoctions are made with roots and dried berries. Infusions are made by bringing water almost to a boil, pouring it over herbs in a cup or teapot, and letting it steep ten to fifteen minutes depending on desired strength. Decoctions need a little more time for the active principles to be released and are often simmered on the lowest setting for an hour after the water has been brought to a boil.

Attracting Love Tisane

- ½ part red rose petals
- ½ part pink rose petals
- ½ part jasmine flowers
- ½ part lavender flowers

Mix the ingredients together while focusing on finding the perfect partner for you. Put the tea in a tea ball or other steeping device and steep the infusion for ten minutes in hot water. Drink at least once a day until you find love.

Clairvoyance Tisane

- 1 part chamomile flowers
- 1 part mugwort
- 1 part cinnamon
- ¼ part orange rind

Mix all the ingredients together and steep the infusion in hot water for ten minutes. Strain the herbs and add sweetener as needed.

Deep Sleep Tisane

- 1 part hops
- 1 part lavender flowers
- 1 part jasmine flowers

- 1 part kava
- ½ part valerian root

Mix all the ingredients together and steep the infusion in hot water for twenty minutes. Strain the herbs and add sweetener as needed.

Meditation Tisane

- 1 part agrimony
- 1 part wild lettuce
- 1 part lemon balm
- ½ part valerian root

Mix all the ingredients together and steep the decoction in hot water for twenty minutes. Strain the herbs and add sweetener as needed.

Relaxation Tisane

- 1 part skullcap
- 1 part chamomile
- 1 part lemon balm

Mix all the ingredients together and steep the infusion in hot water for ten minutes. Strain the herbs and add sweetener as needed.

High Priest Tisane

- 1 part vervain
- 1 part eyebright
- 1 part sage
- 1 part mugwort

Mix all the ingredients together and steep the infusion in hot water for ten minutes. Strain the herbs and add sweetener as needed.

High Priestess Tisane

- 1 part mugwort
- 1 part rose petals
- 1 part catnip

Mix all the ingredients together and steep the infusion in hot water for ten minutes. Strain the herbs and add sweetener as needed.

Initiation Tisane

- 1 part blue vervain
- 1 part eyebright
- 1 part mugwort
- 1 part peppermint

Mix all the ingredients together and steep the infusion in hot water for ten minutes. Strain the herbs and add sweetener as needed.

Tisane to Improve Sexuality

- 1 part damiana
- 1 part yohimbe bark
- 1 part maca
- 1 part lavender flower

Mix all the ingredients together and steep the decoction in hot water for twenty minutes. Strain the herbs and add sweetener as needed.

Salves

Salves are healing ointments. When salves are applied, herbal combinations are absorbed through the skin. Olive oil is a preferred oil to use if the goal is for the salve to penetrate the skin. Both recipes contain beeswax, but vegans can substitute shea butter for the beeswax. Just know that the salve will be thinner.

Healing Salve

- 1 part plantain leaf
- 1 part comfrey leaf
- 1 part yarrow
- 1 part Saint John's wort
- 2 cups of olive oil
- Beeswax to thicken

Using your stove top's lowest setting, simmer the herbs in the oil for at least two hours. Let the herbs cool, then strain them from the oil. Reheat the oil on low and add the beeswax. Once the beeswax has melted, take the oil off the heat and pour it into containers. Use this salve on minor cuts and bruises.

Flying Ointment

- 1 part vervain
- 1 part wild lettuce
- 1 part poppy seeds
- 1 part mugwort
- 2 cups of hemp oil
- Beeswax to thicken

Simmer the herbs and oil in a Crock-Pot overnight on low heat. Cool the oil. Strain the herbs, reheat the oil in a dedicated saucepan, and add beeswax until you reach your desired consistency. Pour the oil into containers. Put flying ointment on pulse points, such as your carotids (neck), underarms, groin (crease between groin and leg), and behind the knees. *CAUTION: This ointment can be toxic when used. Wash your hands after applying it so you don't accidentally ingest it. Wear gloves when preparing it.*

Appendix
MAGICAL ASSOCIATIONS

Angels, communication with

- Angelica
- Cedar
- Jasmine
- Mugwort
- Rose
- Sweetgrass
- Vervain

Angels, to see

- Angelica
- Clary sage
- Eyebright
- Mugwort

Astral Projection

- Cedar
- Mugwort
- Ragweed

- Rattlesnake master
- Vervain

Courage
- Agrimony
- Borage
- Mullein
- Poke
- Yarrow

Court Cases, to win
- Agrimony
- Calendula
- Ground ivy
- Oak

Curses, to protect against
- Angelica
- Datura
- Galangal
- Holly
- Huckleberry
- Lady's mantle
- Osha root
- Poke
- Tansy
- Thistle
- White sage

Divination
- Camphor
- Clary sage
- Dandelion flowers
- Eyebright
- Ground ivy

- Meadowsweet
- Rue
- Yarrow

Dreams, prophetic

- Angelica
- Betony
- Clary sage
- Mugwort
- Yarrow

Employment

- Ground ivy
- Orange
- Pecan
- Walnut

Fertility

- Banana
- Daffodil
- Dock
- Fig
- Hawthorn flowers
- Hazel
- Mandrake
- Nuts
- Passionflower
- Patchouli
- Pine
- Pomegranate
- Poppy
- Sunflower

Gossip, to stop

- Adder's-tongue
- Agrimony
- Clove
- Slippery elm

Grounding

- Burdock
- Dandelion root
- Dock
- Oak

Happiness

- Catnip
- Hawthorn berry
- Lavender
- Lemon balm
- Meadowsweet
- Passionflower
- Saint John's wort

Healing

- Allspice
- Angelica
- Bay
- Benzoin
- Burdock
- Camphor
- Cedar
- Cinnamon
- Dock
- Elder
- Eucalyptus
- Fennel
- Frankincense

- Garlic
- Ginseng
- Goldenseal
- Ground ivy
- Henna
- Horehound
- Mint
- Mullein
- Myrrh
- Nettle
- Oak
- Peppermint
- Pine
- Plantain
- Potato
- Rose
- Rosemary
- Rowen
- Saint John's wort
- Sandalwood
- Spearmint
- Tansy
- Tobacco
- Vervain
- Violet
- Walnut
- Willow

Hexes, to remove

See Curses

Infertility, to create

- Pomegranate rind
- Tansy

- Wild carrot
- Wormwood
- Yarrow

Infertility, to remove

- Chaste tree berries
- Daffodil
- Damiana
- Fig
- Hazel
- Mandrake
- Nuts
- Passionflower
- Pine nuts
- Pomegranate seeds
- Poppy
- Trillium

Infidelity

- Camphor
- Chaste tree berries (for men)
- Cinnamon
- Deer's-tongue
- Ginseng
- Mandrake
- Nettle
- Saw palmetto berries (for men)

Invisibility

- Angelica
- Betony
- Chicory
- Clary sage
- Fern, royal

- Heliotrope
- Mistletoe

Love

- Apple
- Basil
- Betony
- Catnip
- Chamomile
- Cinnamon
- Cleavers
- Clove
- Coca
- Copal
- Coriander
- Daffodil
- Daisy
- Damiana
- Elm
- Fern, maidenhair
- Fern, male
- Fig
- Gardenia
- Ginseng
- Hemp
- Hibiscus
- High John or galangal root
- Jasmine
- Kava
- Lady's mantle
- Lavender
- Lemon balm

- Linden
- Lotus
- Mandrake
- Maple
- Mastic
- Meadowsweet
- Mimosa
- Nuts
- Orchid
- Peppermint
- Plumeria
- Poppy
- Primrose
- Rose
- Rosemary
- Rue
- Skullcap
- Spearmint
- Sweetgrass
- Tulip
- Valerian
- Vanilla
- Vervain
- Violet
- Willow
- Yohimbe

Loyalty

- Agrimony
- Cypress
- Lavender
- Lemon balm
- Sage
- Oak

Luck

- Agrimony
- Allspice
- Daffodil
- Fern, maidenhair
- Fern, male
- Hazel
- Holly
- Irish moss
- Linden
- Lucy hand (orchid root)
- Nutmeg
- Oak
- Orange
- Poppy
- Rose
- Star anise
- Violet

Lust, to decrease

- Camphor
- Chaste tree berries
- Saw palmetto berries
- Vervain
- Wild lettuce

Lust, to increase

- Cinnamon
- Daisy
- Damiana
- Deer's-tongue
- Dill
- Galangal
- Garlic
- Ginseng

- Hibiscus
- Lemongrass
- Mint
- Mugwort
- Nettle
- Patchouli
- Rosemary
- Yohimbe

Meditation

- Benzoin
- Frankincense
- Gotu kola
- Lavender
- Mugwort
- Myrrh
- Patchouli
- Rose
- Sandalwood
- Storax

Money

- Allspice
- Basil
- Bladderwrack
- Cedar
- Chamomile
- Cinnamon
- Cinquefoil
- Comfrey
- Cowslip
- Elder
- Galangal
- Goldenrod
- Heliotrope

- Jasmine
- Mandrake
- Mint
- Nutmeg
- Oak
- Patchouli
- Pine
- Poppy
- Tea
- Vervain
- Woodruff

Obstacles, to overcome

- Agrimony
- Hops
- Horsetail
- Wild geranium

Peace

- Blue vervain
- Daisy
- Lavender
- Lemon balm
- Meadowsweet
- Olive
- Rose
- Violets

Power

- Burdock
- Dragon's blood
- Elecampane
- Horsetail

Prosperity
- Basil
- Benzoin
- Ground ivy
- Jasmine
- Mandrake
- Olive
- Solomon's seal
- Tea

Protection
- Agrimony
- Angelica
- Asafetida
- Blue vervain
- Burdock
- Chamomile
- Dragon's blood
- Elder
- Elecampane
- Frankincense
- Garlic
- Ground ivy
- Holly
- Jewelweed
- Lady's mantle
- Nettle
- Nightshade
- Oak
- Rosemary
- Rue
- Sage
- Saint John's wort
- Solomon's seal
- Valerian

- Wild geranium
- Yarrow

Psychic Abilities, to decrease

- Burdock root
- Lemon balm
- Rosemary

Psychic Abilities, to increase

- Borage
- Calendula
- Celery
- Clary sage
- Dandelion
- Eyebright
- Henbane
- Mugwort
- Peppermint
- Wild yam
- Wood sorrel
- Yarrow

Purification

- Angelica
- Asafetida
- Benzoin
- Blue vervain
- Cedar
- Dandelion
- Dragon's blood
- Frankincense
- Goldenseal
- Juniper
- Meadowsweet
- Mugwort

- Peppermint
- Rosemary
- Rue
- Tobacco
- Wood sorrel
- Yarrow

Sexuality

- Basil
- Burdock
- Catnip
- Celery
- Damiana
- Dragon's blood
- Ginseng
- Henbane
- Mandrake
- Rose
- Wild carrot
- Wild yam
- Yohimbe

Spirituality

- Angelica
- Blue vervain
- Catnip
- Clary sage
- Echinacea
- Jasmine
- Mugwort
- Tobacco
- Valerian (for offerings to cat deities only)
- Wild bergamot
- Wild geranium
- Wild yam

Strength

- Echinacea
- Elecampane
- Hops
- Horsetail
- Mugwort
- Oak
- Plantain
- Rose
- Rosemary
- Tea
- Wild carrot
- Wild geranium

Success

- Basil
- Ground ivy
- Holly
- Horsetail
- Jasmine
- Mandrake
- Nettle

Wisdom

- Echinacea
- Eyebright
- Mugwort
- Sage
- Wild bergamot

Youth

- Lady's mantle
- Lemon balm
- Olive
- Rosemary

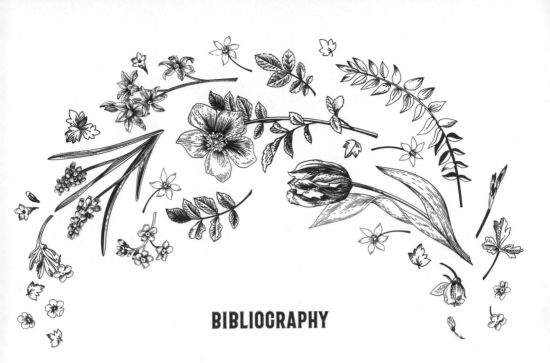

BIBLIOGRAPHY

Agrippa von Nettesheim, Henry Cornelius. *The Philosophy of Natural Magic: A Complete Work on Natural Magic, White Magic, Black Magic, Divination, Occult Binding, Sorceries, and Their Power. Unctions, Love Medicines and Their Virtues*. Secaucus, NJ: University Books, 1974.

Best, Michael R., and Frank H. Brightman, eds. *The Book of Secrets of Albertus Magnus: Of the Virtues of Herbs, Stones, and Certain Beasts, Also a Book of the Marvels of the World*. New York: Oxford University Press, 1973.

Beyerl, Paul. *A Compendium of Herbal Magick*. Custer, WA: Phoenix Publishing, 1998.

———. *The Master Book of Herbalism*. Custer, WA: Phoenix Publishing, 1996.

Blumenthal, Mark, Werner R. Busse, Alicia Goldburg, Joerg Gruenwald, Tara Hall, Chance W. Riggins, and Robert S. Rister, eds. *The Complete German Commission E Monographs: Therapeutic Guide to Herbal Medicines*. Translated by Sigrid Klein and Robert S. Rister. Austin, TX: American Botanical Council, 1998.

Boericke, William. *Pocket Manual of Homeopathic Materia Medica & Repertory*. Delhi, India: Indian Books & Periodicals Publishers, 1999.

Brundage, Albert H. *A Manual of Toxicology: A Concise Presentation of the Principal Facts Relating to Poisons, with Detailed and Descriptive Directions for the Treatment of Poisoning, a Table of Doses of the Principal and Many New Remedies and Various Statistical Tables*. New York: D. Appleton, 1929.

Budge, E. A. Wallis. *Amulets and Talismans*. Toronto: Collier-MacMillan, 1970.

———. *Egyptian Magic*. New York: Dover Publications, 1971.

Centers for Disease Control and Prevention. "Jimson Weed Poisoning—Texas, New York, and California, 1994." *MMWR Morb Mortal Wkly Rep* 44, no. 3 (January 1995): 41–44.

Chaucer, Geoffrey. "The Knight's Tale." In *The Canterbury Tales*, 23–24. Philadelphia: Franklin Classics, 2018.

"Cocktail Medicine: Borage." Food Republic. Accessed May 1, 2023. https://www.foodrepublic.com/2011/07/05/cocktail-medicine-borage/.

Culpeper, Nicholas. *Culpeper's Complete Herbal & English Physician*. Glenwood, IL: Meyerbooks, 1990.

Cunningham, Scott. *Cunningham's Encyclopedia of Magical Herbs*. St. Paul, MN: Llewellyn Publications, 1985.

Eliade, Mircea. *Zalmoxis, the Vanishing God: Comparative Studies in the Religions and Folklore of Dacia and Eastern Europe*. Translated by Willard R. Trask. Chicago: The University of Chicago Press, 1972.

Ellingwood, Finley. *The American Materia Medica, Therapeutics and Pharmacognosy*. Chicago: Ellingwood's Therapeutist, 1919.

Evelyn, John. *The Diary of John Evelyn*. Edited by John Bowle. New York: Oxford University Press, 1985.

Felter, Harvey Wickes, and John Uri Lloyd. *King's American Dispensatory*. Cincinnati: Ohio Valley, 1989.

Fortune, Dion. *The Sea Priestess*. Boston: Weiser Books, 2003.

Galen of Pergamum. *On the Constitution of the Art of Medicine. The Art of Medicine. A Method of Medicine to Glaucon*. Edited and translated by Ian Johnston. Cambridge, MA: Harvard University Press, 2016.

Gerard, John. *The Herbal: Or General History of Plants*. New York: Dover Publications, 1975.

Graves, Robert. *The White Goddess: A Historical Grammar of Poetic Myth*. New York: Farrar, Straus, and Giroux, 1999.

Grieve, M. *A Modern Herbal: The Medical, Culinary, Cosmetic and Economic Properties, Cultivation, and Folk-Lore of Herbs, Grasses, Fungi, Shrubs & Trees with All Their Modern Scientific Uses*. New York: Barnes and Noble, 1996.

Griffin, Judy. *Mother Nature's Herbal*. St. Paul, MN: Llewellyn Publications, 1997.

Griggs, Barbara. *The Green Witch Herbal: Restoring Nature's Magic in Home, Health & Beauty Care*. Rochester, VT: Healing Arts Press, 1994.

Hatsis, Thomas. *The Witches' Ointment: The Secret History of Psychedelic Magic*. Rochester, VT: Park Street Press, 2015.

Hoffmann, David. *The New Holistic Herbal*. Boston: Element Books, 1992.

Hopman, Ellen Evert. *A Druid's Herbal for the Sacred Earth Year*. Rochester, VT: Destiny Books, 1995.

Hutchens, Alma R. *A Handbook of Native American Herbs*. Boston: Shambhala Books, 1992.

Jones, Pamela. *Just Weeds: History, Myths, and Uses*. New York: Prentice Hall Press, 1991.

Krutch. Joseph Wood. *Herbal*. New York: Putnam, 1965.

Leek, Sybil. *Sybil Leek's Book of Herbs*. Nashville: T. Nelson, 1973.

Leland, Charles Godfrey. *Etruscan Magic & Occult Remedies*. New York: University Books, 1963.

———. *Gypsy Sorcery and Fortune Telling: Incantations, Specimens of Medical Magic, Anecdotes, Tales.* New York: Citadel Press, 1990.

Micromedex, Inc. "Belladonna." In *Micromedex Healthcare Series.* Englewood, CO: Thomas Reuters, 2001.

———. "Goldenseal." In *Micromedex Healthcare Series.* Englewood, CO: Thomas Reuters, 2001.

———. "Jimson Weed." In *Micromedex Healthcare Series.* Englewood, CO: Thomas Reuters, 2001.

Meydenbach, Jakob. *Ortus sanitatis.* Mainz, 1491. https://collections.nlm .nih.gov/catalog/nlm:nlmuid-9413026-bk.

Ovid. *Metamorphoses.* Translated by Frank Justus Miller. London: William Heinemann, 1926.

"Pando." USDA Forest Service. Accessed May 1, 2023. https://www.fs.usda .gov/detail/fishlake/home/?cid=STELPRDB5393641.

Paracelsus, Philippus Aureolus. *Hermetic & Alchemical Writings of Paracelsus the Great.* The Alchemical Press, 1992.

Pliny the Elder. *Natural History: A Selection.* Translated by John F. Healy. New York: Penguin Books, 1991.

Porta, Giambattista della. *Natural Magick.* The Collector's Series in Science. New York: Basic Books, 1957.

Riddle, John M. *Dioscorides on Pharmacy and Medicine.* Austin, TX: University of Texas Press, 1985.

Rose, Jeanne. *Herbs & Things: Jeanne Rose's Herbal.* New York: Perigee Books, 1972.

Saint Hildegard. *Hildegard von Bingen's Physica: The Complete English Translation of Her Classic Work on Health and Healing.* Translated by Priscilla Throop. Rochester, VT: Healing Arts Press, 1998.

Scott Walter, ed. Hermetica: *The Ancient Greek and Latin Writings which Contain Religious or Philosophic Teachings Ascribed to Hermes Trismegistus.* Boston: Shambhala, 1985.

Scudder, John M. *Specific Medication and Specific Medicines*. Cincinnati: Wilstach, Baldwin & Co., 1870.

Valiente, Doreen. *Natural Magic*. New York: St. Martin's Press, 1975.

Wissler, Clark, and D. C. Duvall, trans. *Mythology of the Blackfoot Indians: Sources of American Indian Oral Literature*. Lincoln, NE: University of Nebraska Press, 1995.

Wood, Matthew. *The Book of Herbal Wisdom: Using Plants as Medicine*. Berkeley, CA: North Atlantic Books, 1997.

To Write to the Author

If you wish to contact the author or would like more information about this book, please write to the author in care of Llewellyn Worldwide Ltd. and we will forward your request. Both the author and the publisher appreciate hearing from you and learning of your enjoyment of this book and how it has helped you. Llewellyn Worldwide Ltd. cannot guarantee that every letter written to the author can be answered, but all will be forwarded. Please write to:

Aurora
℅ Llewellyn Worldwide
2143 Wooddale Drive
Woodbury, MN 55125 2989

Please enclose a self-addressed stamped envelope for reply,
or $1.00 to cover costs. If outside the U.S.A., enclose
an international postal reply coupon.

Many of Llewellyn's authors have websites with additional information and resources. For more information, please visit our website at http://www .llewellyn.com.